Dani Goes to Fabry Family Camp

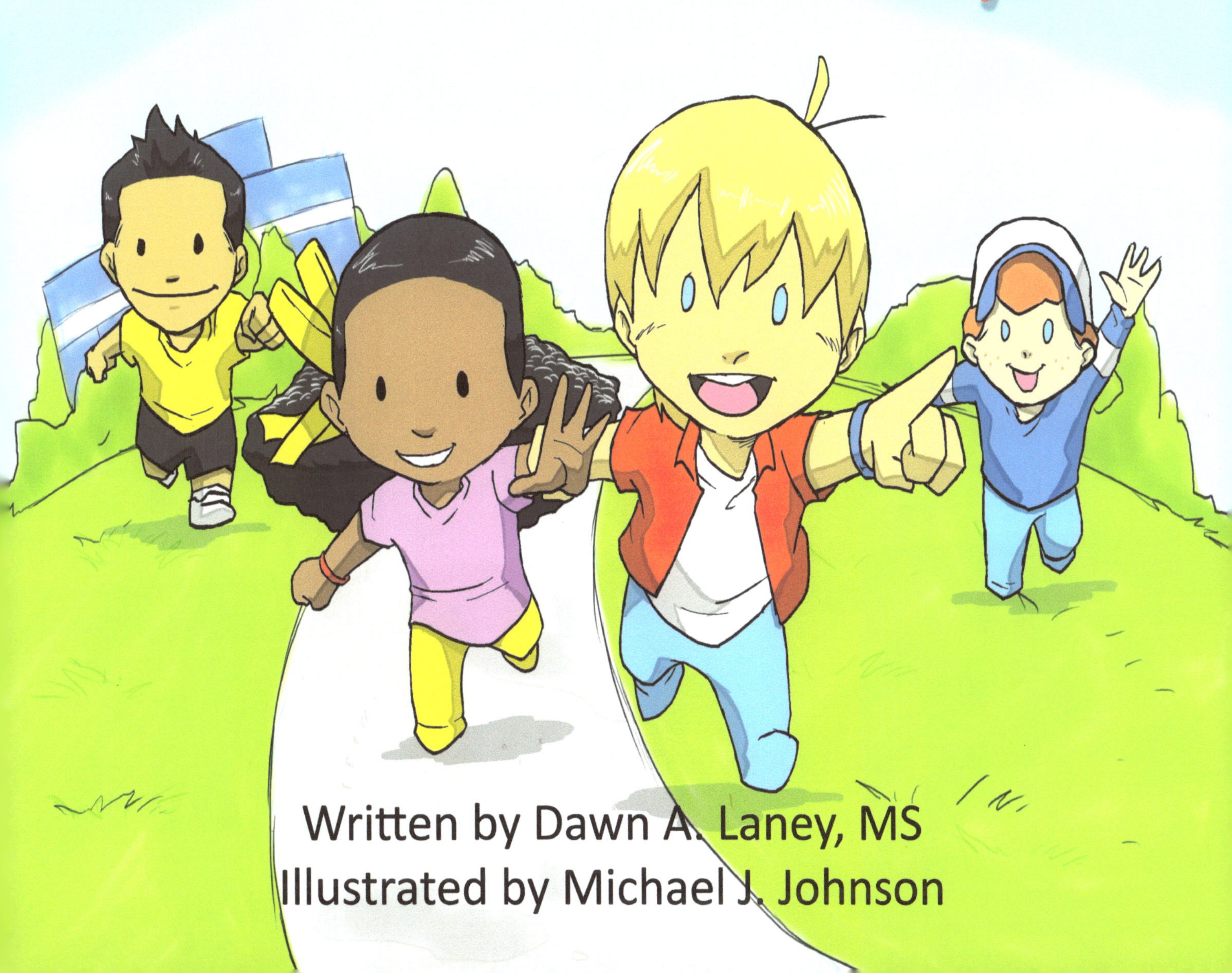

Written by Dawn A. Laney, MS
Illustrated by Michael J. Johnson

Copyright © 2014 Dawn A. Laney
All rights reserved

ISBN-13: 978-1492887645
ISBN-10: 1492887641

With thanks to Jerry Walter, Angela Walter, & Jack Johnson who support us all.

Dani was nervous. She had butterflies bumping and thumping all around in her stomach. She and her parents were about to board a plane to Fabry Family Camp. The plane wasn't the problem- she liked flying. The butterflies were flying because she was both excited and a little scared to go to camp.

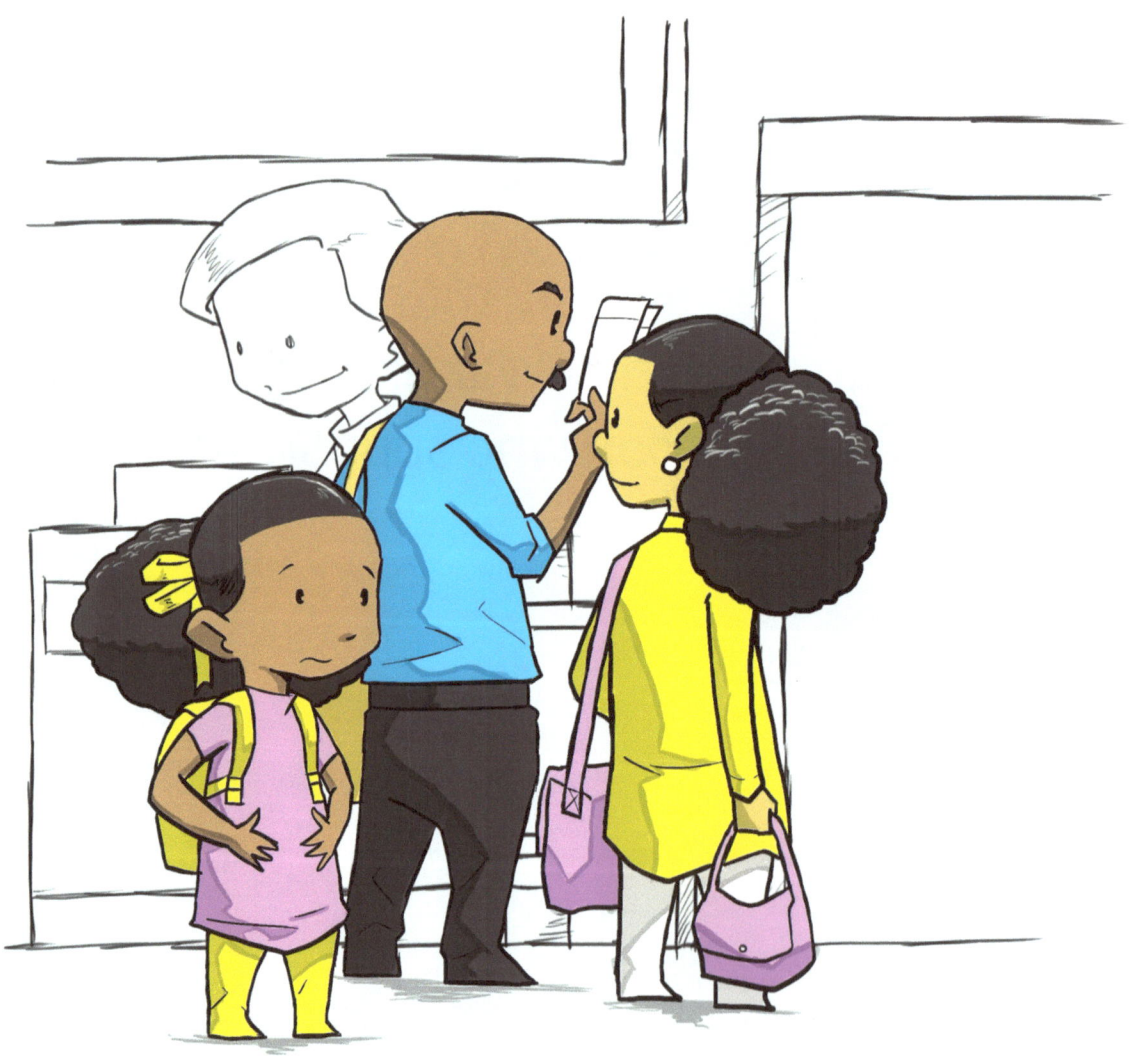

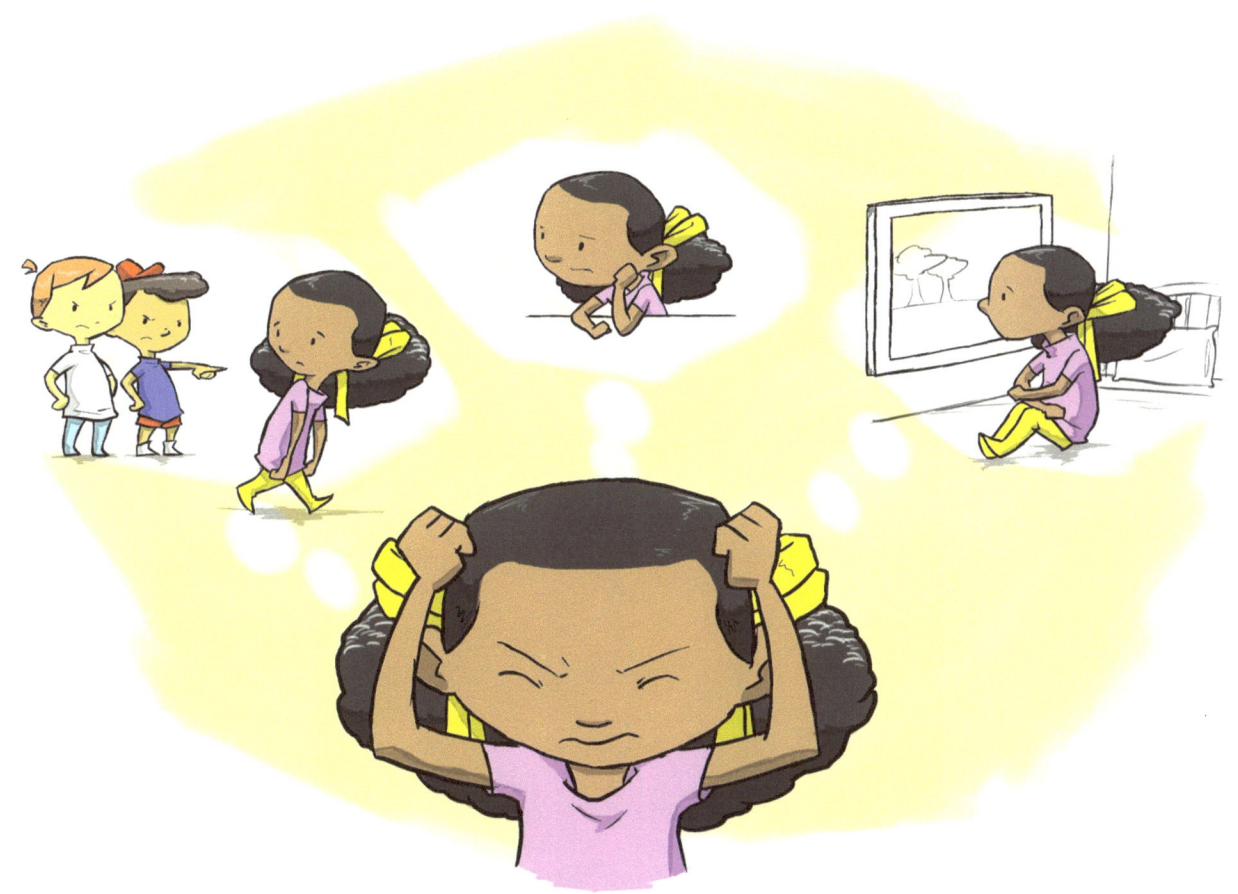

What if the other kids didn't like her? What if camp was boring? What if her stomach acted up and she had to stay inside her cabin, missing all the fun? Dani's parents kept telling her that it would all be ok, that it WOULD be fun to meet other kids who were living with Fabry disease. They told her the other kids would totally understand if she got too hot, her feet hurt, or she had to get to the bathroom FAST. Dani didn't know any other kids with Fabry disease, just her dad and uncle, and they were adults. It was hard for her to picture a whole CAMP of kids and parents with Fabry disease.

As she was thinking, the gate agent made the boarding announcement for her zone. There were a lot of people standing by the gates with baggage. Dani and her parents patiently moved through the crowd, gave the gate agents their boarding passes, headed down the jet way, and moved into their seats.

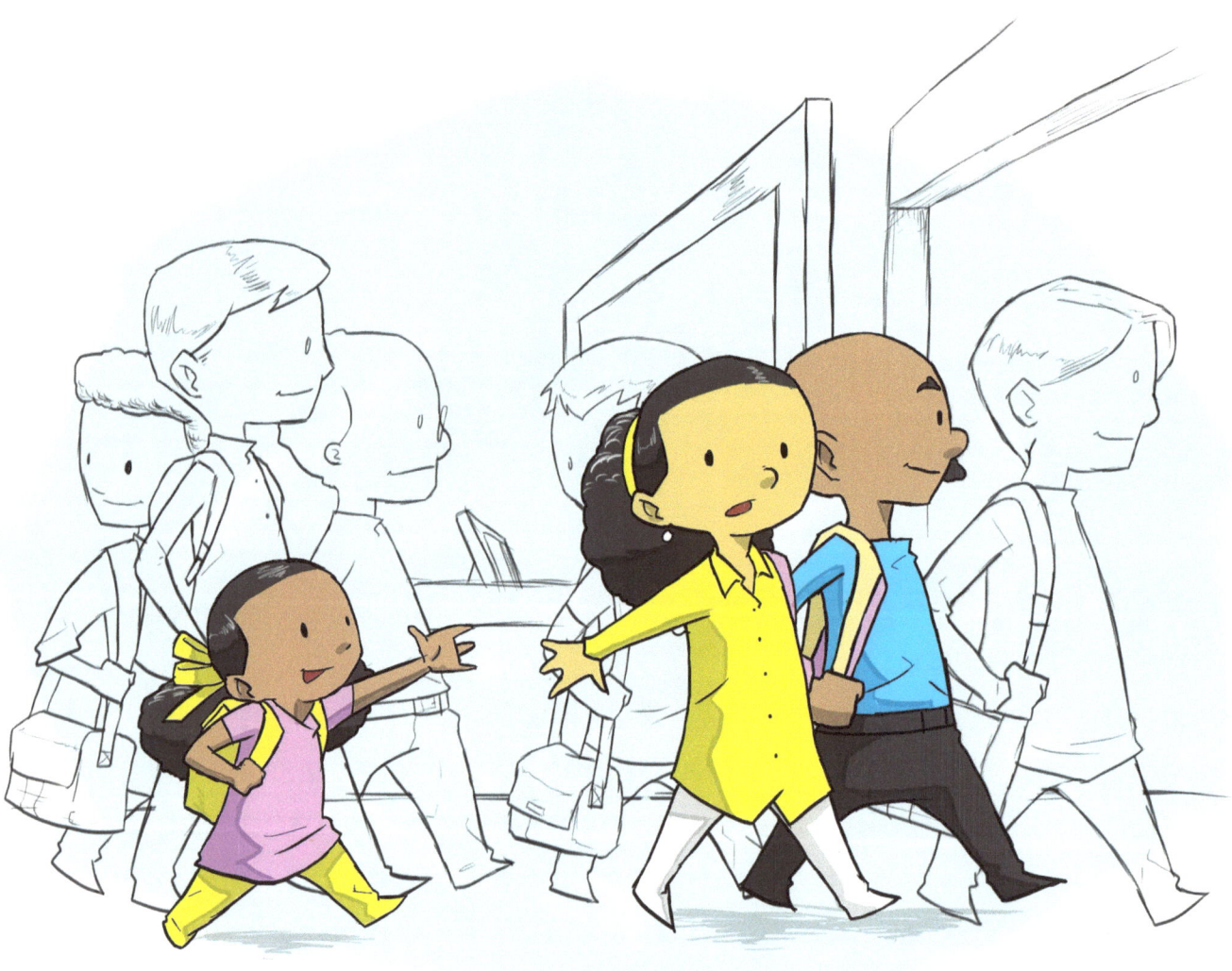

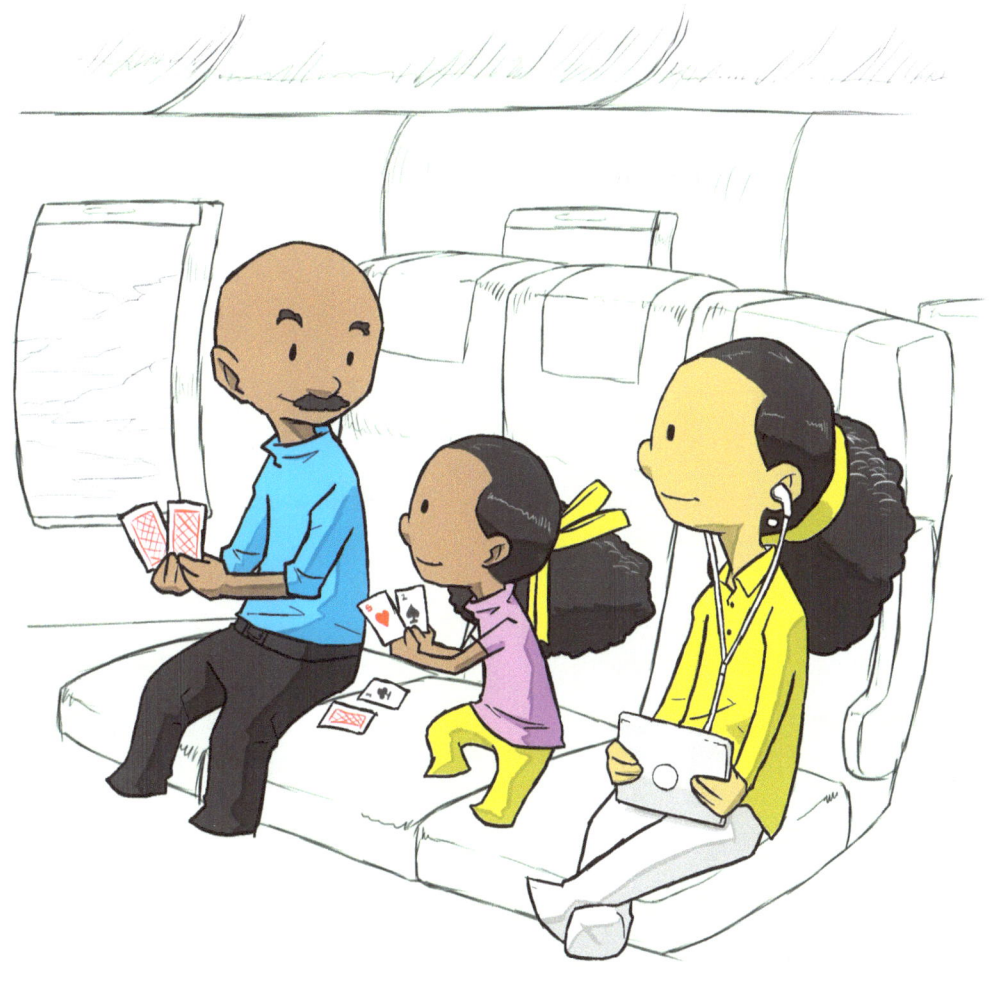

The flight was fun, but a little long. Dani read her book, played cards with her dad, and watched a movie on her mom's iPad. Finally they landed and headed out to get their bags.

As they were waiting for their luggage, Dani's mom took a close look at her face. "Dani?" she said, "How's your stomach? You look a little pale." Dani gave a small smile. "I'm not so bad, Mom. Just a little...nervous."

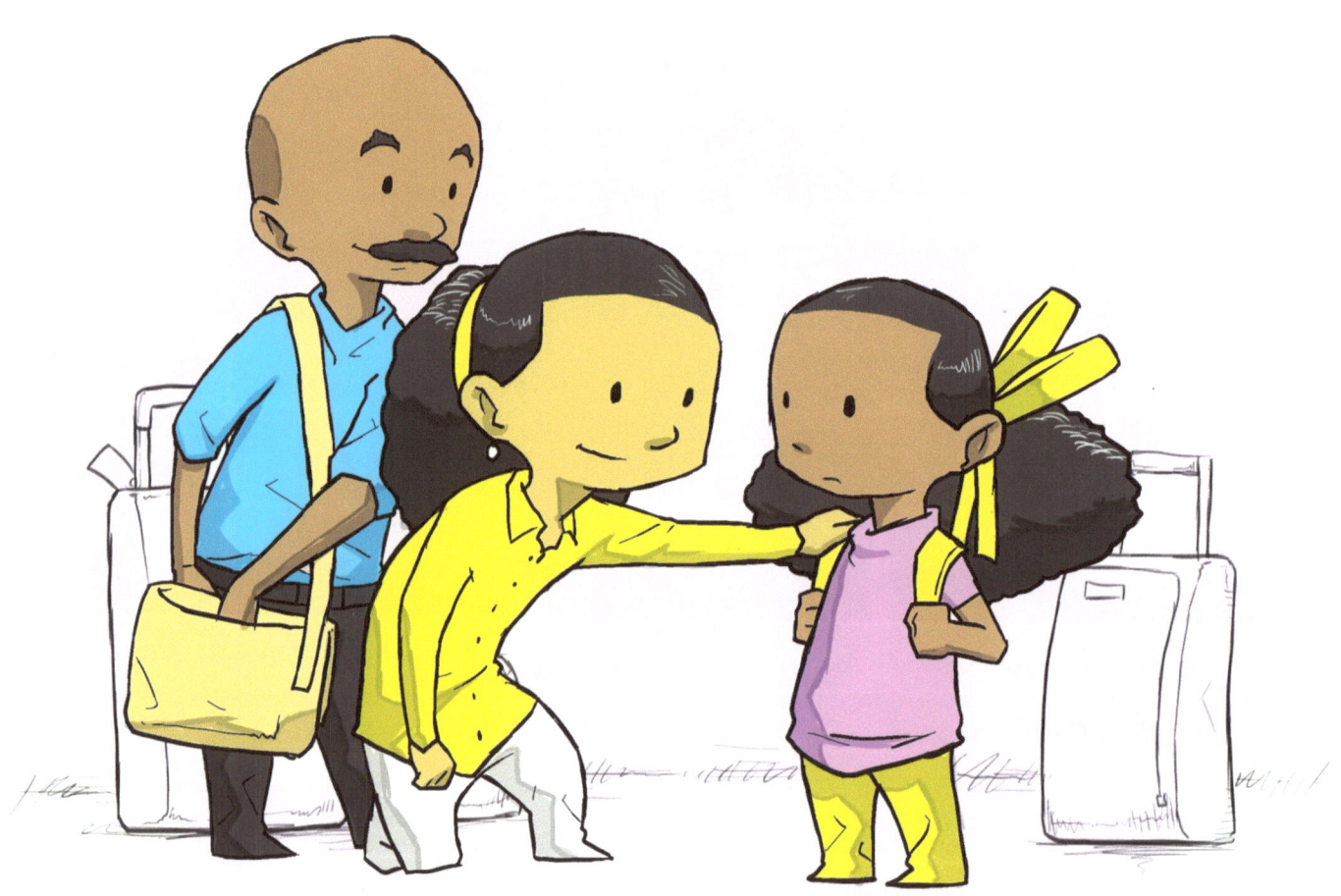

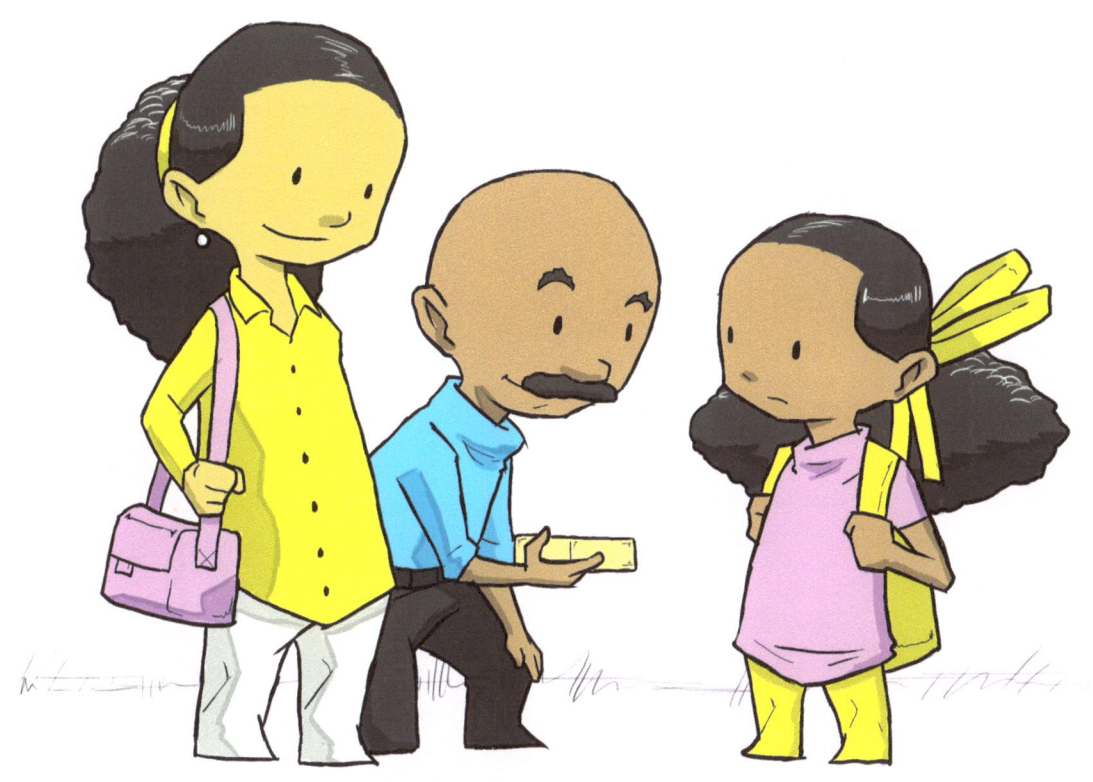

Both her parents smiled at her and her dad said, "I know this is a completely new thing and new things can be scary, but we'll all be there together. Tell you what, we were going to wait to give you this until later, but your mother and I think giving it to you now might help you feel a little less worried." Dani's dad handed her a small box with a bright blue bracelet with yellow words and a red bracelet with white words on it.

The blue bracelet said "Fighting Fabry Disease" in yellow. "Sounds like a plan," thought Dani. The red bracelet, read, "Fabbers helping Fabbers." She smiled to herself, Fabber was a funny word, but she got it. Fabber was a cute nickname for someone with the same condition she had: someone living with Fabry disease.

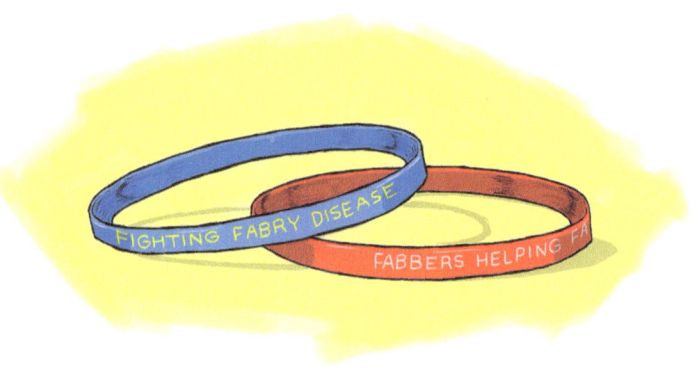

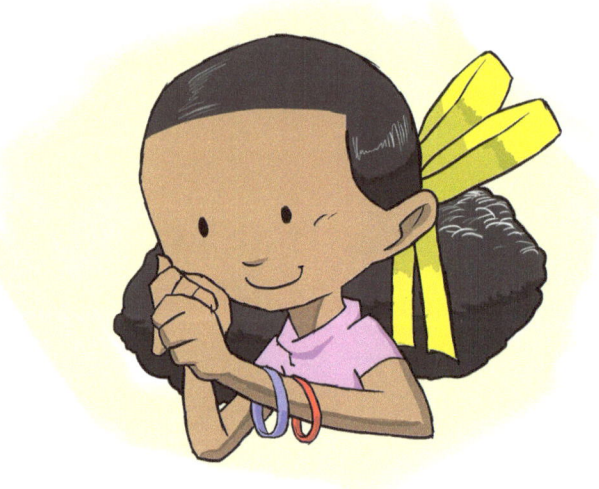

Dani's mom said, "We thought these bracelets would help remind you that we're heading to a camp filled with people just like you. The whole point of camp is for everyone to meet each other and have fun together." Dani slipped the bracelets on her wrist. Her belly butterflies settled down a little. The bracelets were a great reminder that this camp was for her!

Even so, Dani's butterflies began to flutter a little bit as she and her parents got on the big camp bus and saw other families with kids.

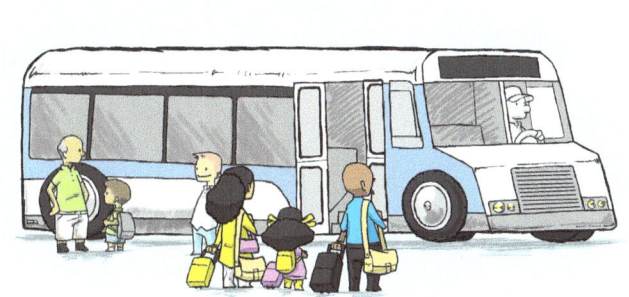

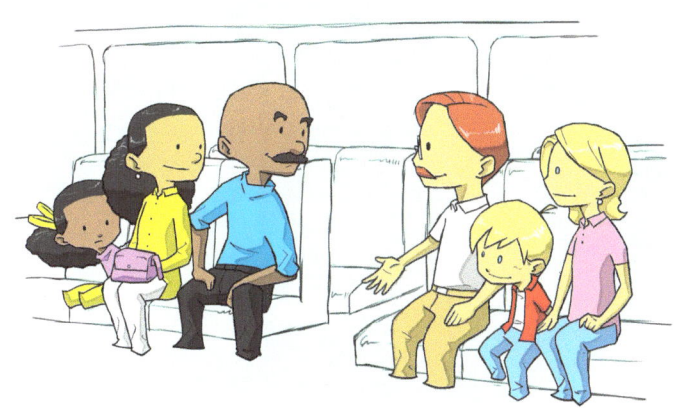

As they rode the bus, Dani's parents introduced themselves to the family sitting next to them. Dani peered around her mother to look at the boy with them. She noticed that he had the same bracelets she did. Her dad made the introduction, "Dani, this is Joe. He has Fabry disease too!"

Joe smiled broadly at Dani, "Hey! Is this your first time at camp?" Joe asked. Dani gave a shy smile and nodded her head. "Cool!" said Joe, "It's my third time. Want me to show you around?" Dani was a little unsure, but her mom gently nudged her and said, "Go ahead Dani, your dad and I will unpack and settle in. We'll meet up at the dining hall if you don't make it back to the cabin before dinner."

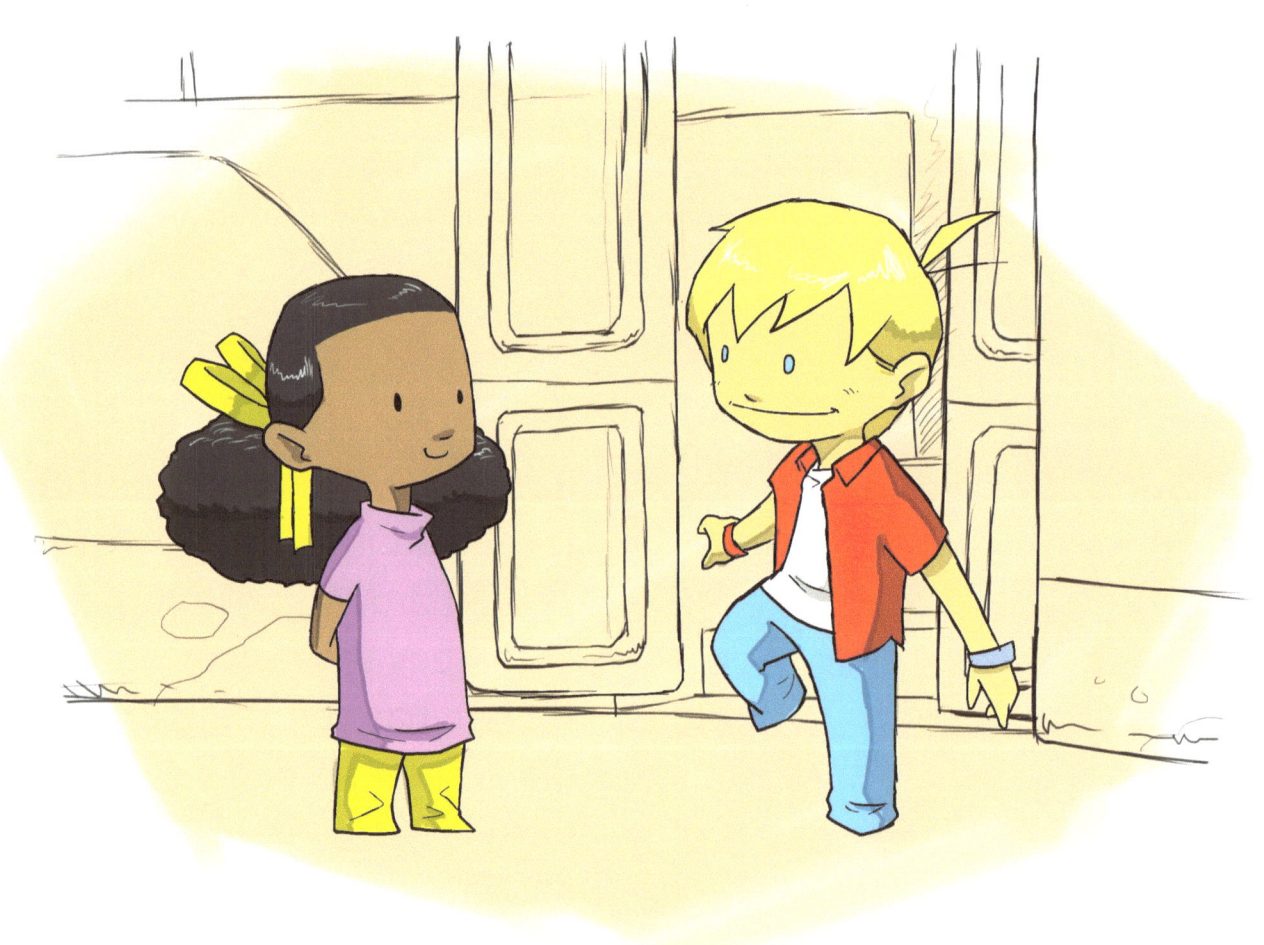

Joe was an excellent tour guide. He knew all the short cuts from place to place. He also seemed to know everyone! He said hi and introduced her to each person saying, "This is Dani. It's her first time at camp."

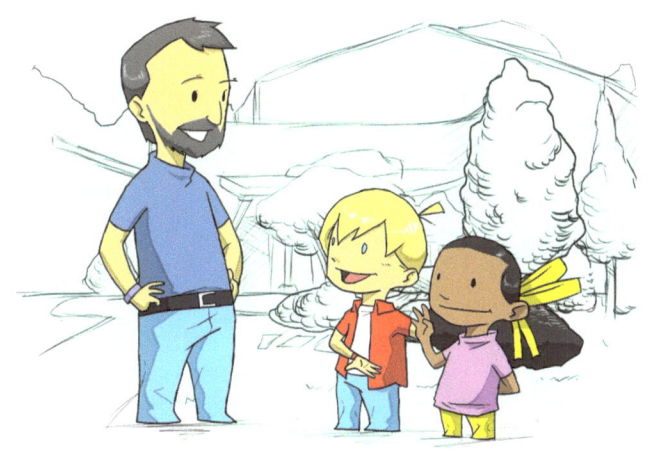

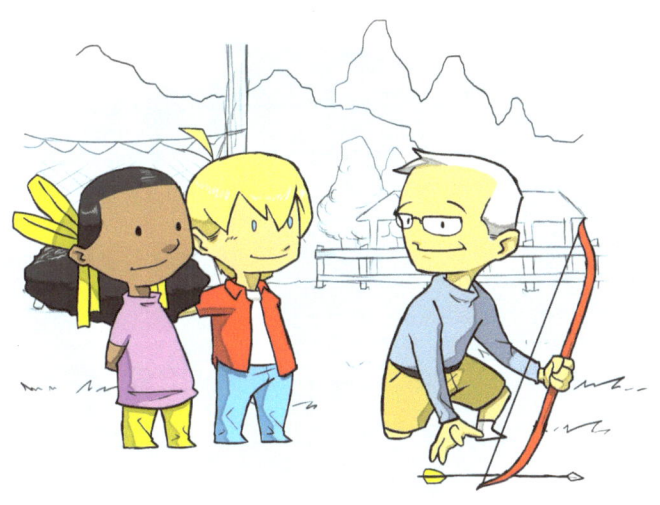

After each person moved on, he told Dani a little bit about them. "Oh! That's Larry, he is a volunteer who runs the archery area. He's great!" or "That's Dr. H, he's cool! He comes every year and wanders around answering questions about Fabry disease."

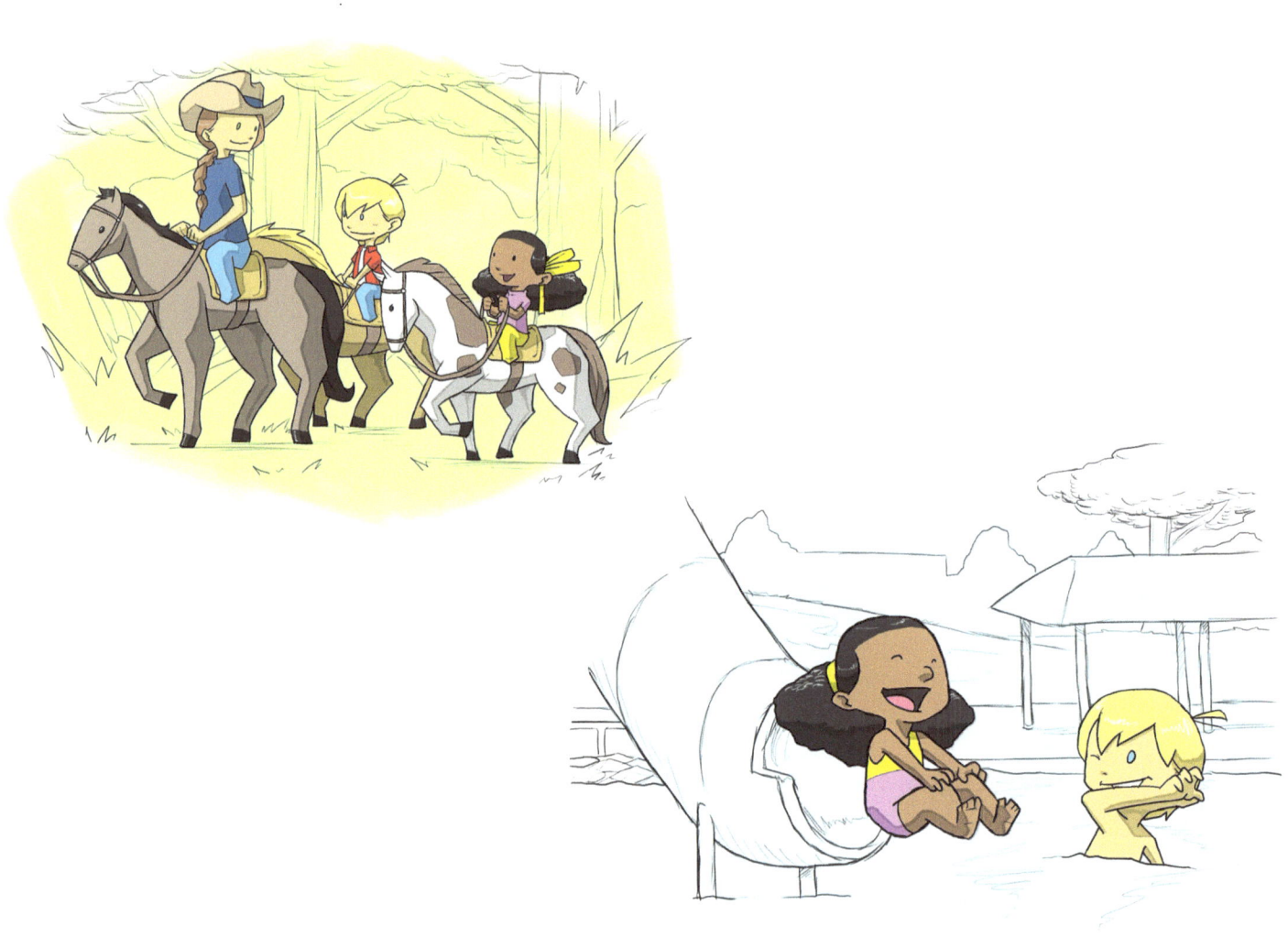

The camp was full of exciting things to do: a pool with water slides, horses to ride, mini golf to play, a stage to perform upon, and even a beauty shop in which to make funny hair styles and do face painting. Dani began to feel more comfortable the more she learned about the camp. She could see herself having a lot of fun here.

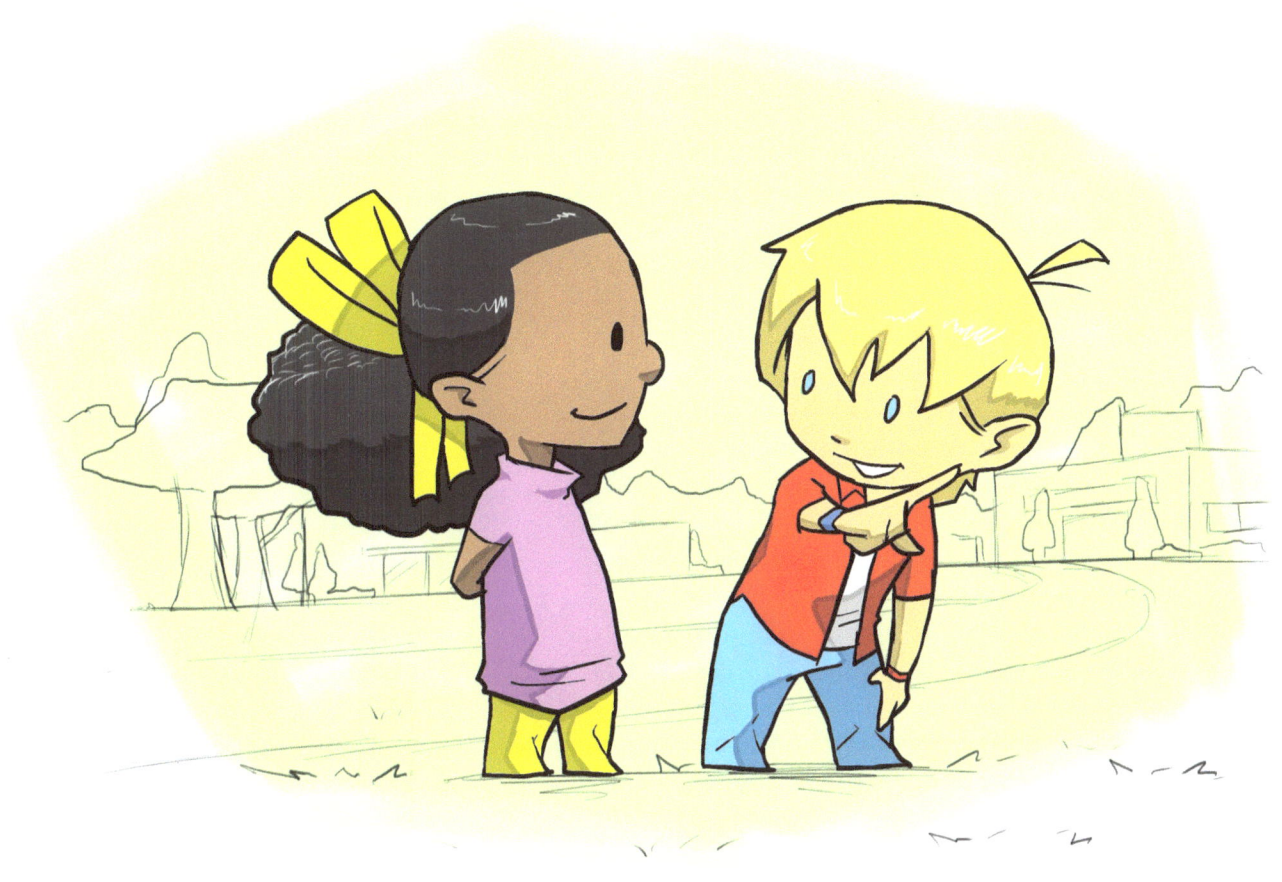

As she and Joe headed past a playing field, Joe said, "Hey, I don't know about you, but I'm getting a little tingly in the feet. Want to go get a snack and sit inside for a minute?" Dani thought that was a great idea and they headed inside.

After getting a cold glass of water and a piece of fruit, the two new friends sat down to talk a little more about camp and life in general. They also watched various people pass by the dining room windows while Joe kept up a running commentary. "That's Jerry and Angela, they are amazing! They organize camp for us every year." or "That's one of the genetic counselors from Georgia, she comes up just for the weekend to be one of our counselors." As they passed, everyone gave Joe and Dani a cheery wave and a smile.

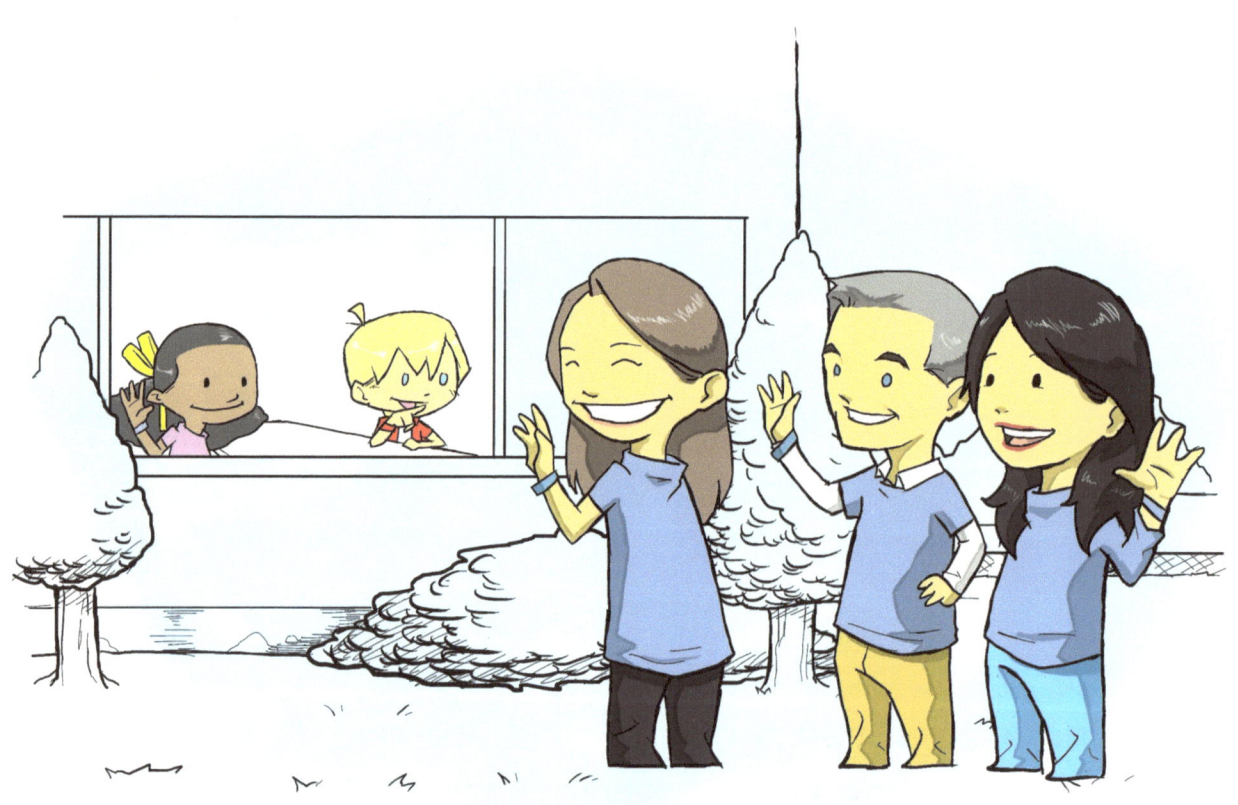

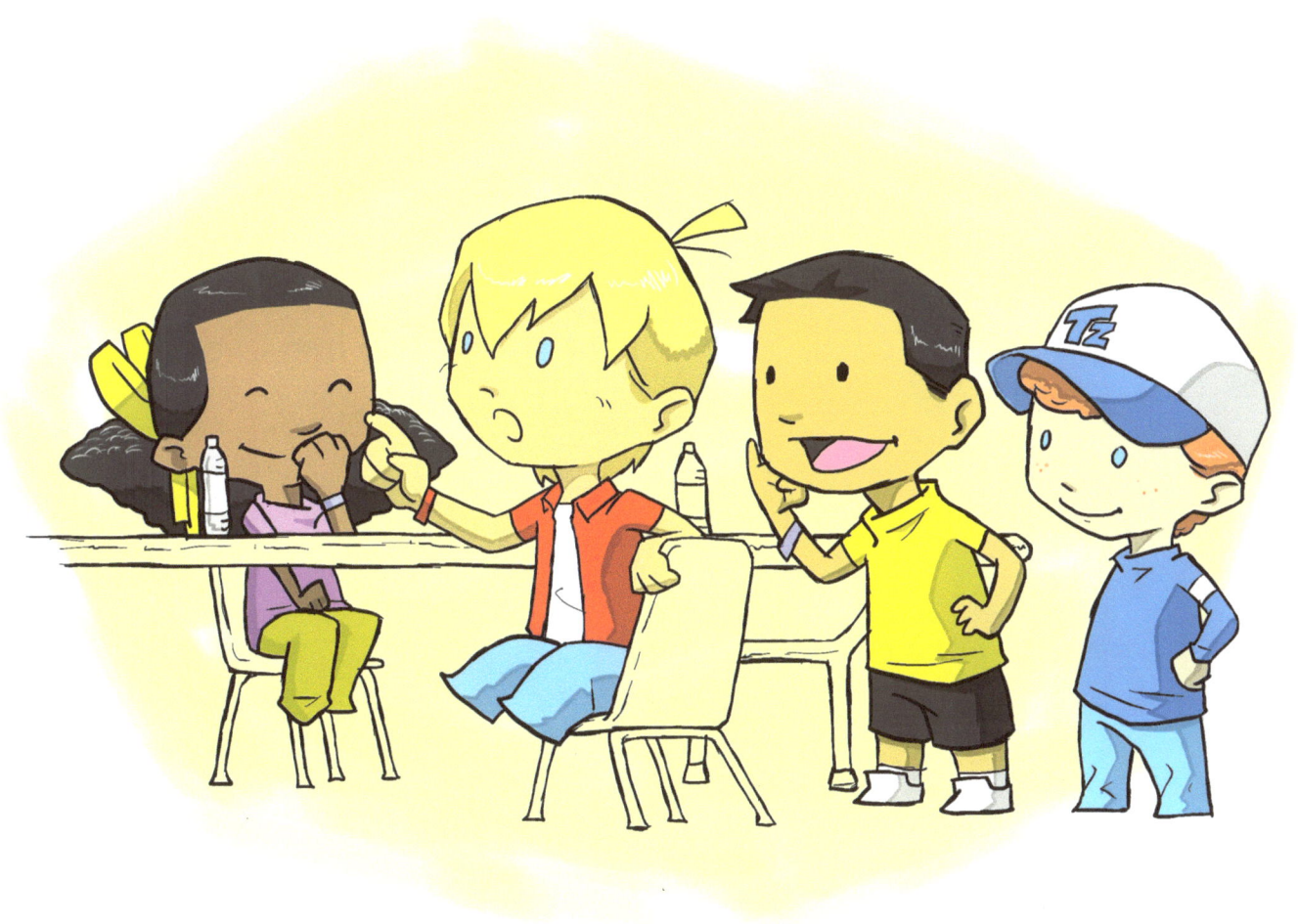

Joe and Dani were so engrossed in their conversation and watching people pass by the window, that they were surprised when two boys came up to say "Hi!".

"Hey Joe!" said one of the guys.

"Hey Aaron!" said Joe, "How's it going? This is Dani. It's her first time at camp."

"Hi Dani, " said Aaron, his brown eyes sparkling. "This is my new friend Robbie. It's his first time here too. "

Dani smiled at the two guys, "Hey," she said, "nice to meet you!"

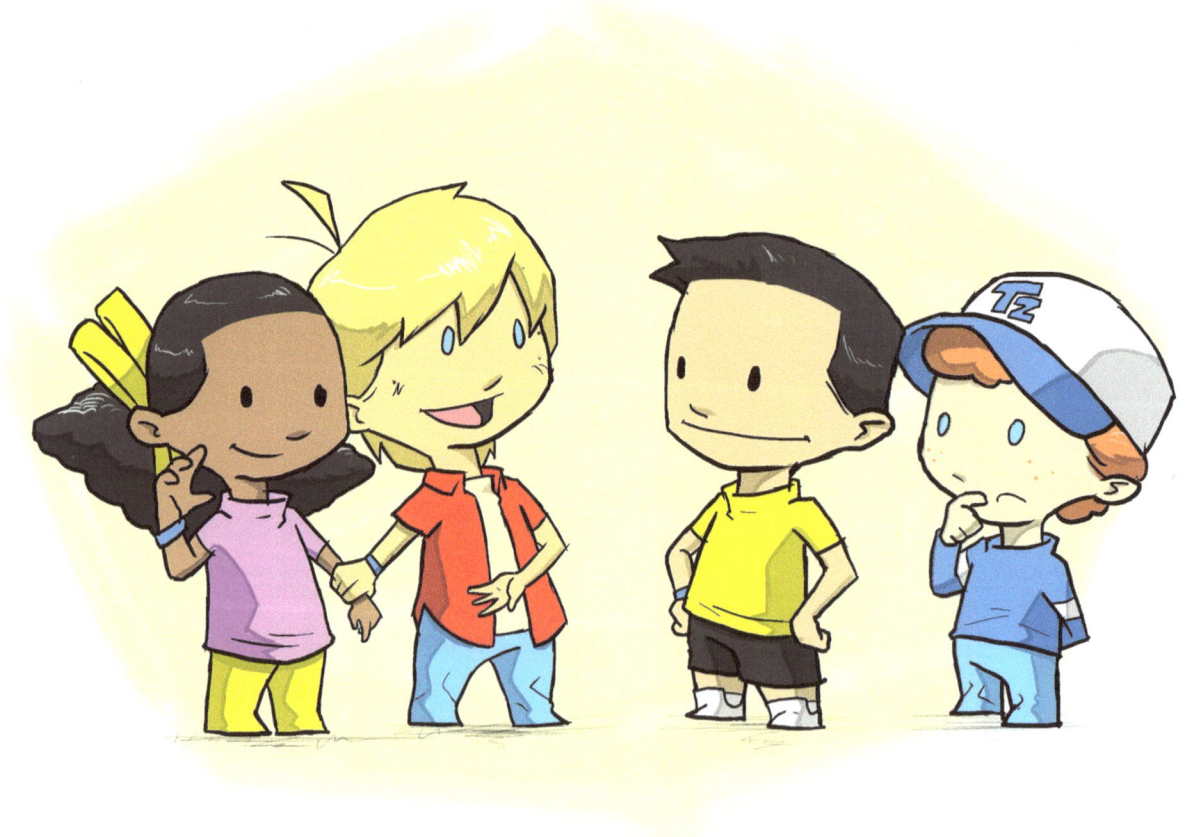

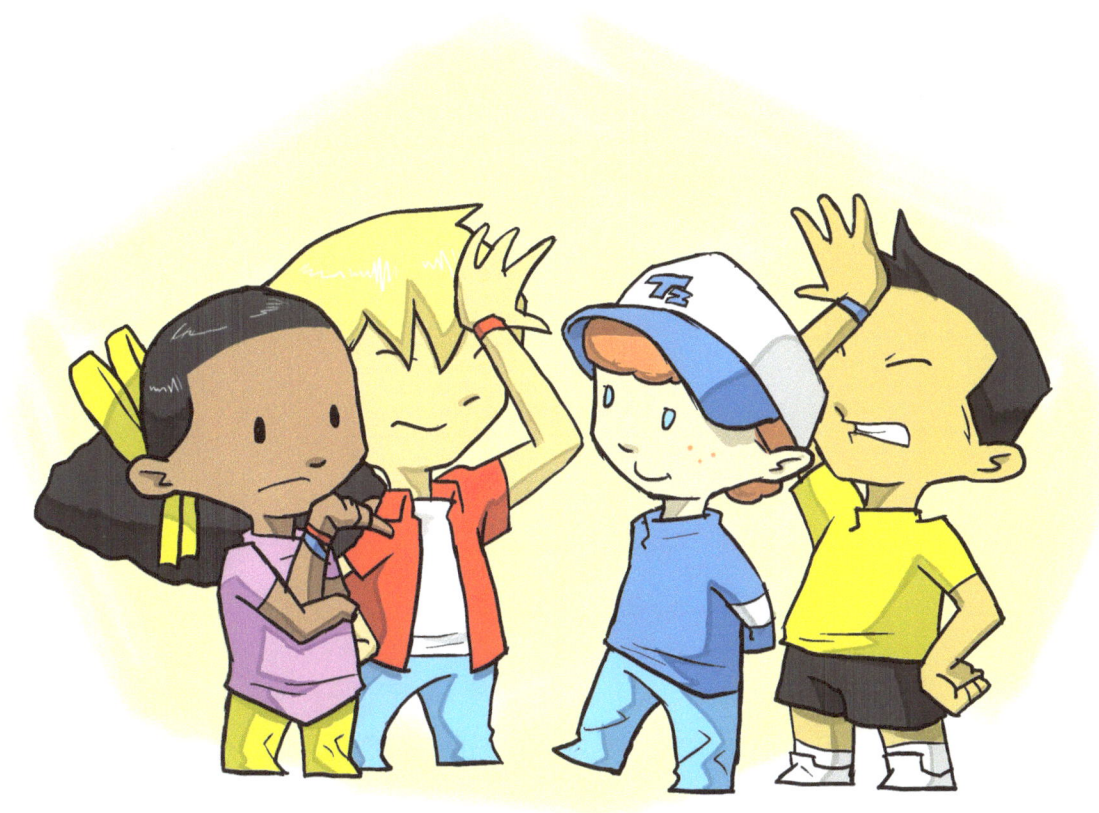

Robbie smiled at Dani, but looked a little puzzled. "Are you here because your brother has Fabry disease?" Robbie asked.

Dani looked at Robbie a little confusedly, "No, I'm an only child. I'm here because I have Fabry disease. Don't you have Fabry disease too?"

Robbie furrowed his forehead, "Sure, I do, but I thought girls couldn't have Fabry disease."

"DUDE!" said Aaron and Joe together.

Aaron continued, "Ahhh…Robbie, I think someone told you some old news. They didn't used to think girls had Fabry disease, but when they really looked, they found that girls have symptoms just like boys."

"Yep," said Joe, "In fact my mom found out that she had Fabry disease just before we figured out that I had it too. My burning feet and tiredness were just like hers."

Robbie, a little embarrassed, looked at Joe and Aaron and said "For real?"

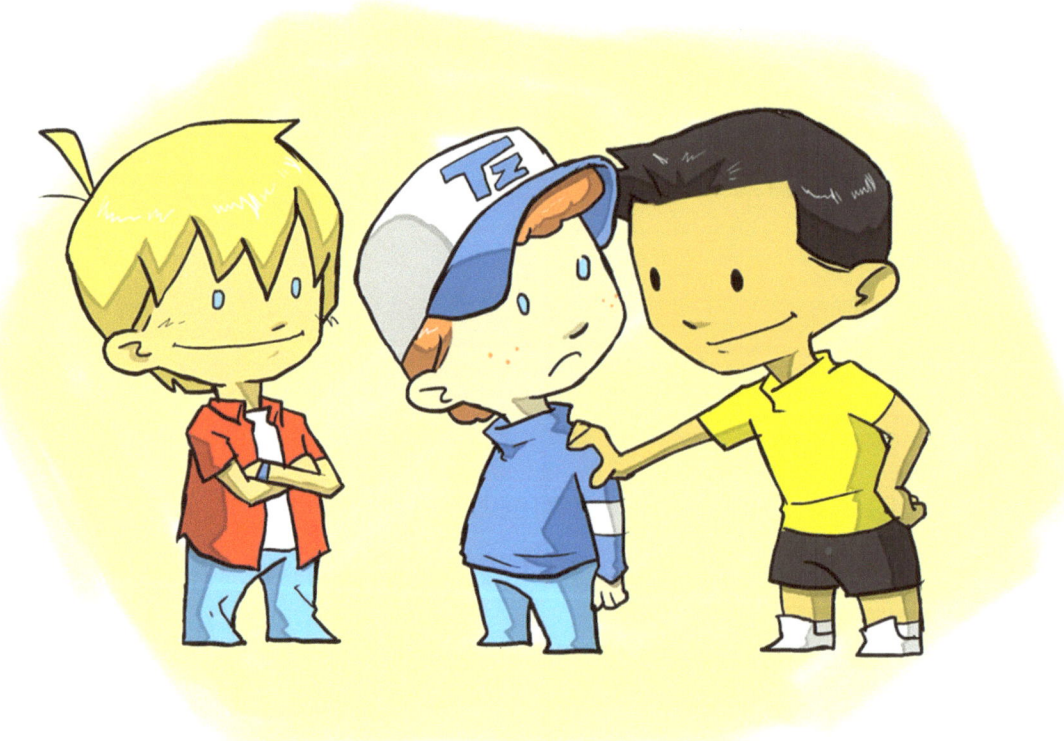

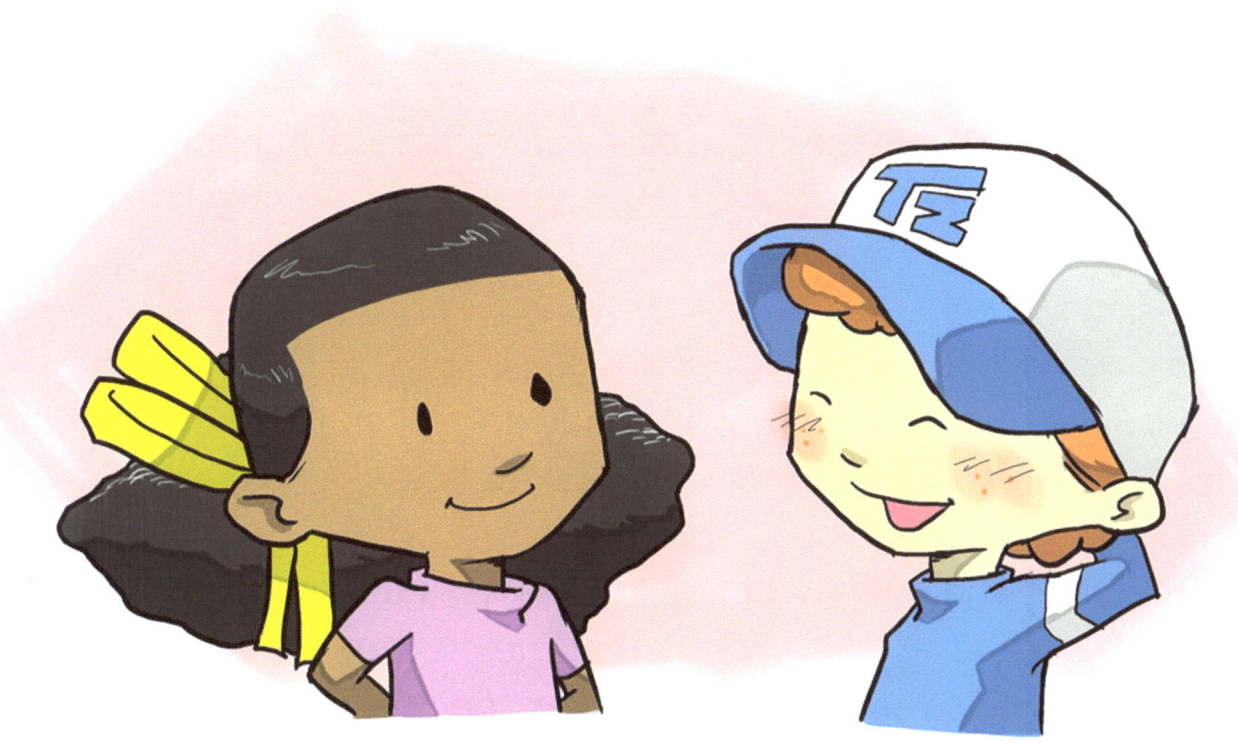

"Oh yeah!" Aaron said, "You'll meet a lot of girls with Fabry this weekend at camp. I'm glad we could clear that up for you now. Of course, there will be lots of brothers and sisters without Fabry disease here too, so never assume one way or the other. "

"Oh!" said Robbie apologetically, "I feel a little silly. Sorry Dani!"

"Don't worry about it,' said Dani. She felt very happy that she had Aaron and Joe there to explain all this to Robbie. She wasn't sure if she could have done it alone.

"Ok, guys," said Robbie, "What else should I know before I say something stupid again?"

Aaron laughed, "Well, you know that Fabry disease happens when your body is missing a certain chemical or enzyme called alpha-gal, right?"

"Kinda." said Robbie.

"Well it is," said Aaron. "When your body doesn't make enough alpha-gal, gunk called GL-3 builds up in the cells of your body."

Joe chimed in, "The buildup of gunk in the cells of your body causes your blood vessels to be smaller. For us that means foot pain, purple freckles, upset stomach, no sweating, and makes us sooo tired sometimes."

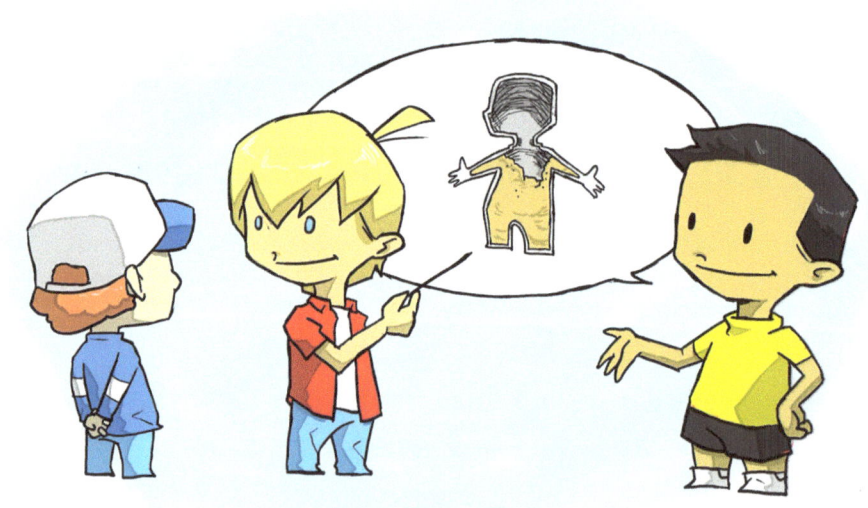

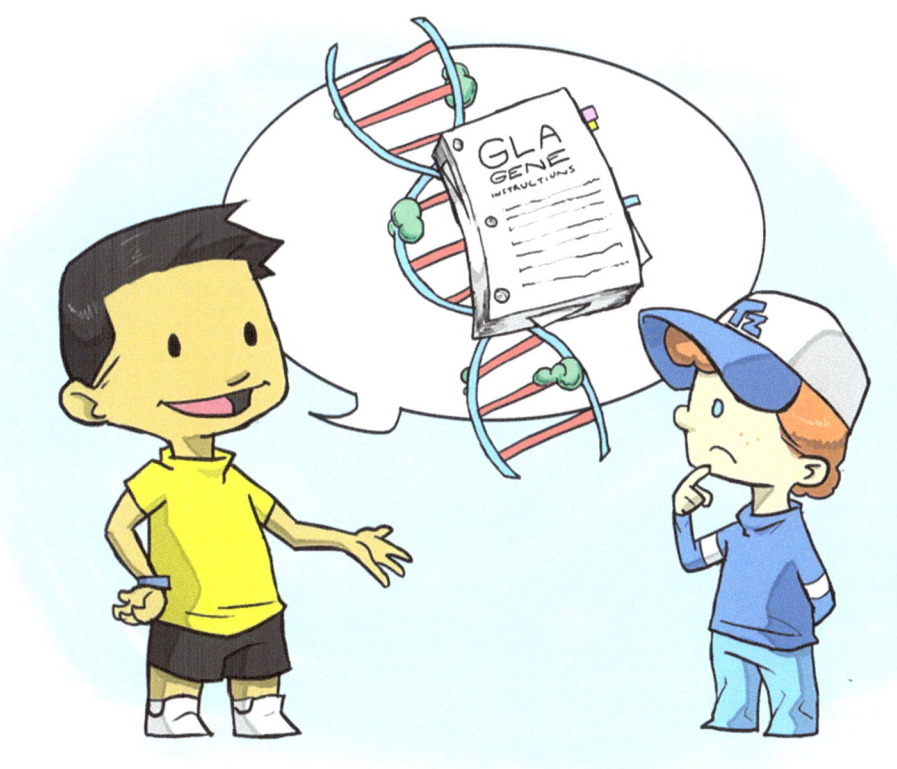

"Why don't our bodies make enough alpha-gal?" asked Robbie.

"Great question!" said Aaron "It's because we have a change or mutation in our GLA gene. The GLA gene has the instructions for making alpha-gal. Changed instructions equal not enough alpha-gal."

Joe then added, "In most people with Fabry disease, the changed GLA gene was passed on from one of their parents."

"Hmmmm…I don't know my dad, " said Robbie, "Did I get it from him?"

"No. Here's the funny thing… " said Aaron, "The GLA gene is on the "X" chromosome. Boys have one "X" chromosome and one "Y" chromosome. Girls have 2 "X" chromosomes.

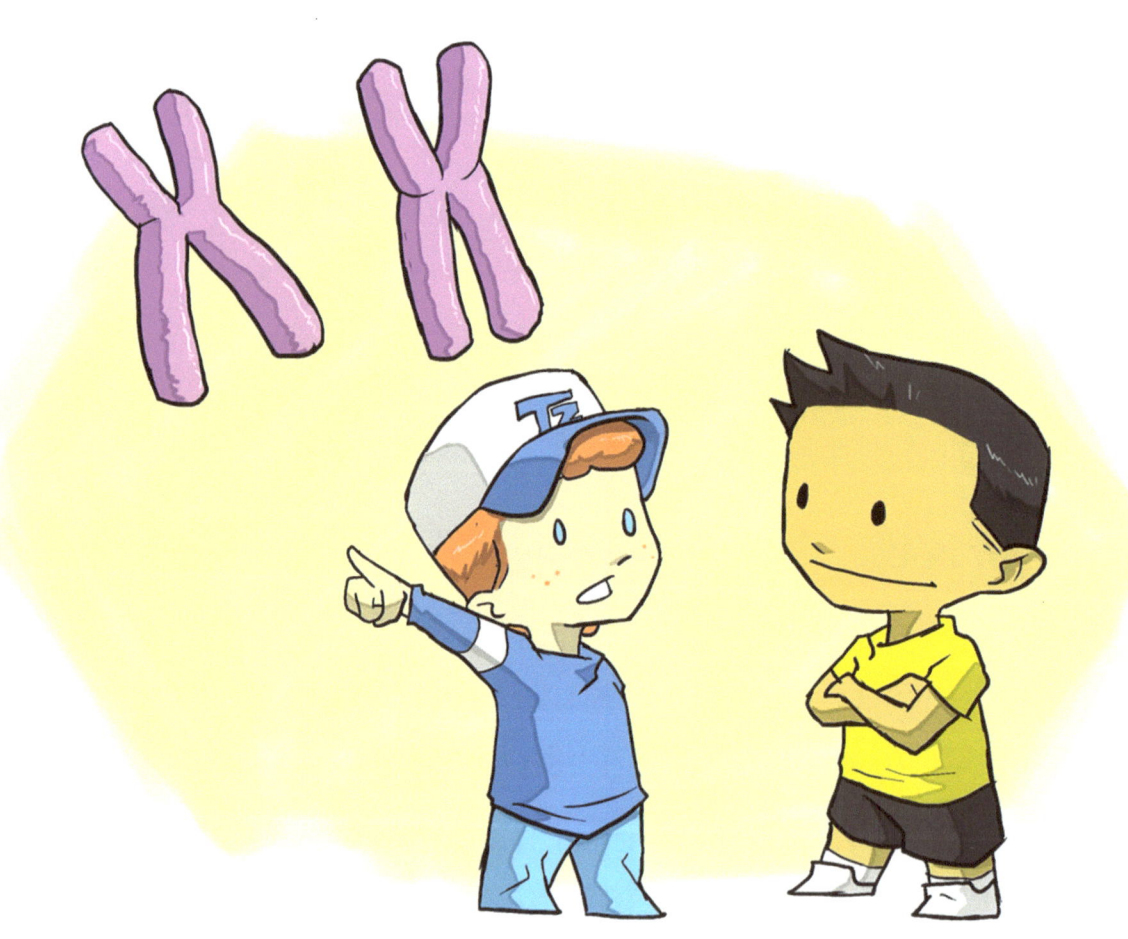

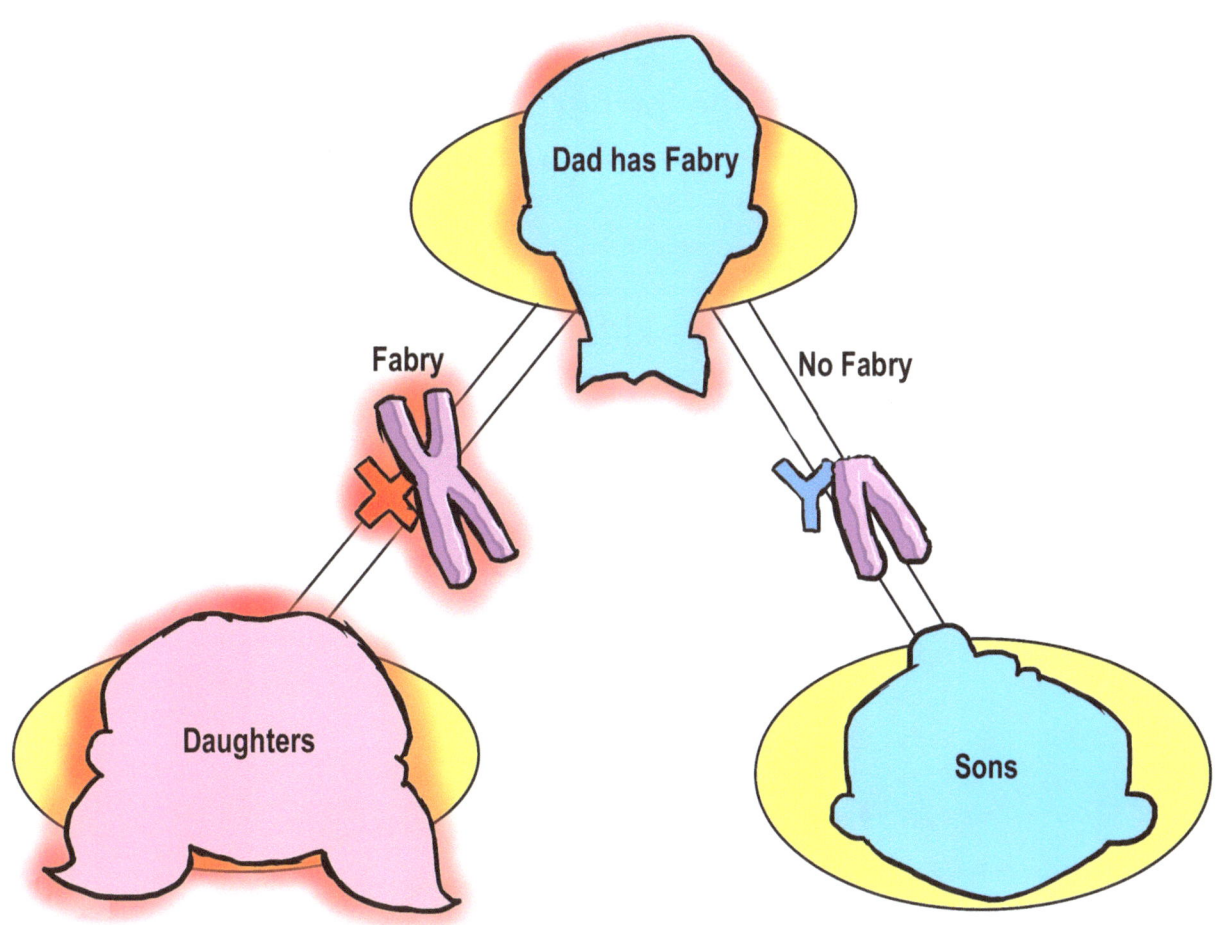

"When a baby is made, the dad either passes on his "X" or his "Y". If he passes on his "Y" he makes a boy. Since the GLA gene isn't on the "Y", a father can't pass on Fabry to his sons. If a dad with Fabry disease passes on his "X", then he makes a girl. Since he only has one "X" and it causes Fabry disease, then ALL of his daughters will have Fabry disease."

"Whoa…" said Robbie, "that's weird!"

"Right?" said Joe, "What's even weirder is that all girls have 2 "X"s, so if a mom has Fabry disease, only one of her X's has the changed GLA gene. Whether she has a daughter or a son, it's a 50% chance for each of her kids to have Fabry disease."

"Ok…" said Robbie, "So, when I have kids, then none of my sons would have Fabry disease, but all of my daughters would…right?"

"Yes!" said Aaron and Joe together.

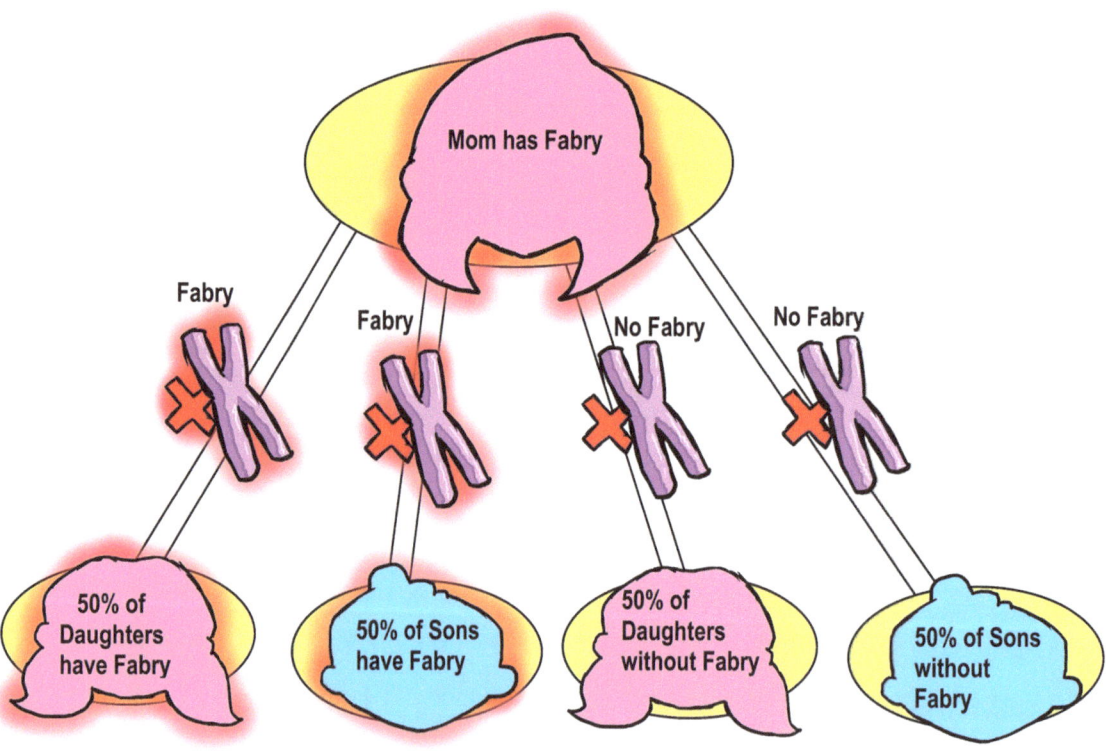

"And if I have kids," said Dani, "it's like flipping a coin. Fifty percent chance for Fabry disease whether it's a boy or a girl."

"You got it!" said Joe, "High fives all around for the Fantastic Fabber Four!"

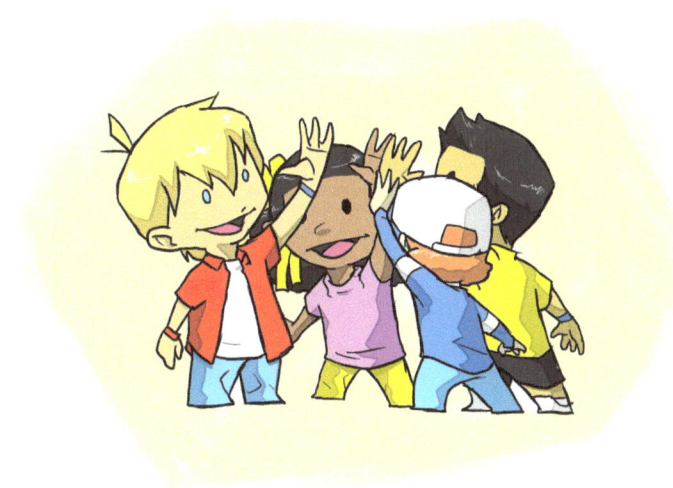

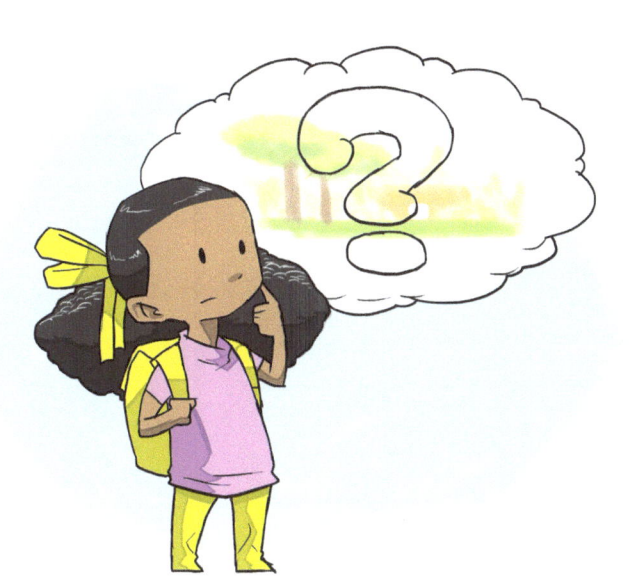

"Wait," said Dani, "I've always wondered this. Can I choose which X to pass on when I have a kid?"

"Nope," said Aaron, "You can't choose which X you pass on, just like Robbie couldn't pick whether he would have a son or a daughter."

"I just wish I could choose when to have my enzyme replacement infusions!" said Aaron. "I feel so worn out after my infusion that I go straight to sleep."

"Do you still get the shakes?" asked Joe.

"Naw, did you ever get them? " asked Aaron.

"Nope, never got the shakes." said Joe "Oh! Did I tell you? My doctor sped up my infusions. They are taking only about 2 hours now."

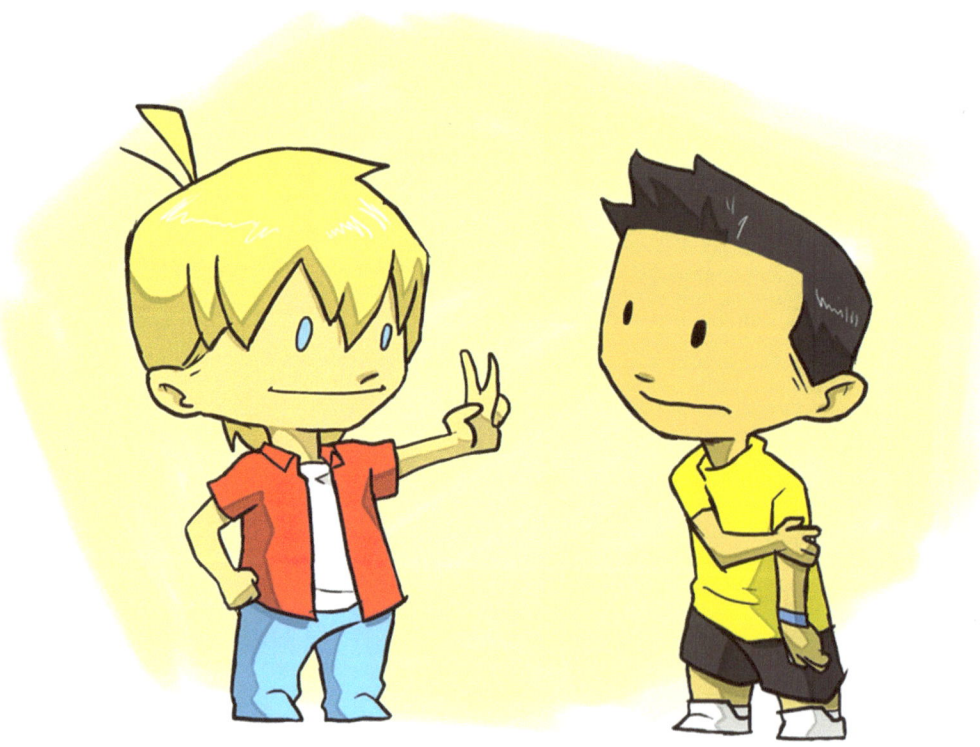

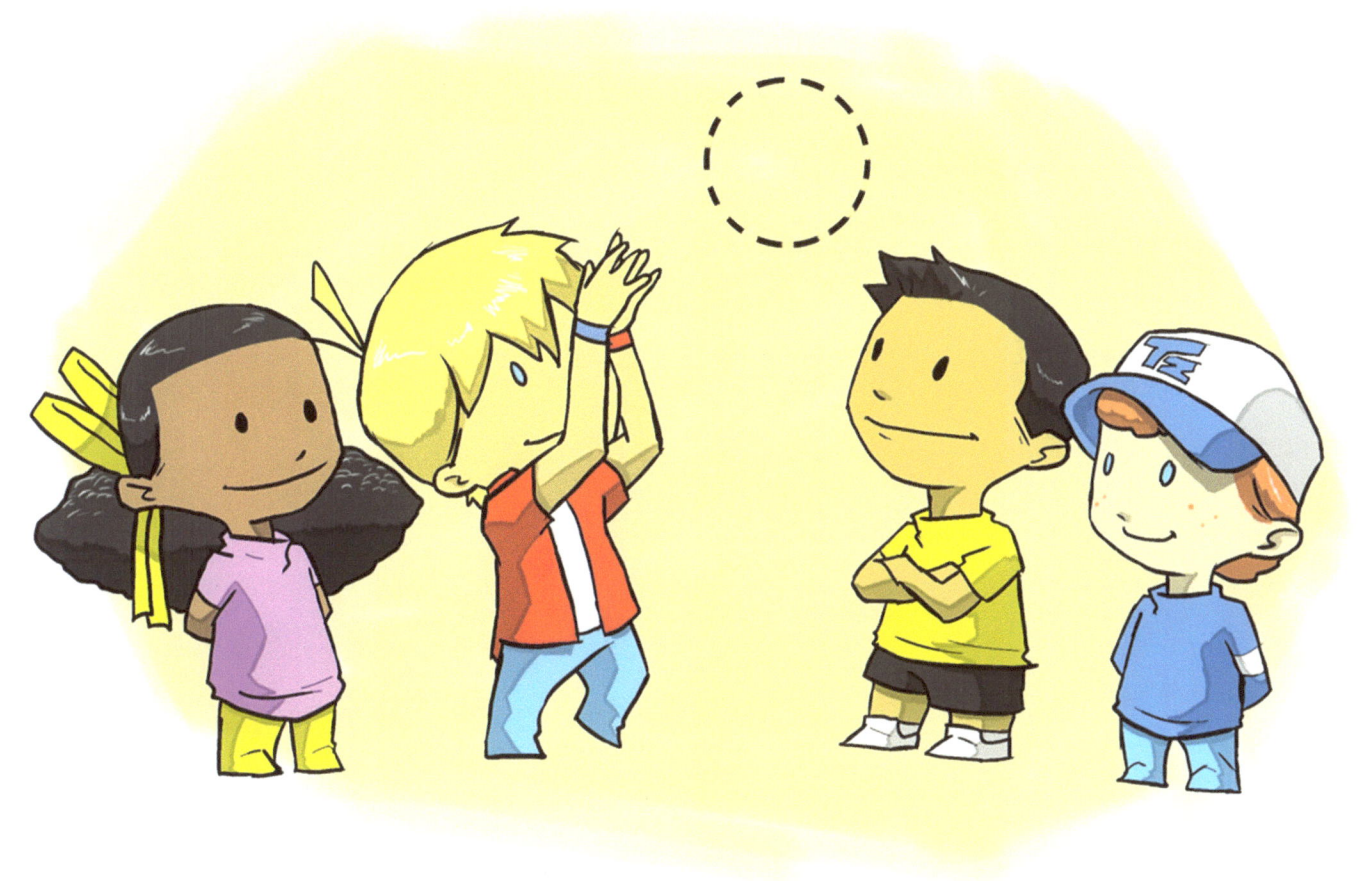

"My feet still hurt, "said Aaron. "I wish they would stop."

"I hear you," said Joe, "I take a pill twice a day to help with my foot pain. Now I really only get tingling in my feet when I'm hot or sick. Although if I'm playing sports and ignore the tingling, the burning will come. It is so much better than it used to be."

"I'm not on infusions," said Robbie, "should I be?"

"Probably, but you need to ask your doctor." said Aaron, "My mom says that even though Enzyme Replacement Therapy infusions aren't a cure, they help clear the GL3 gunk out of our cells. The earlier your start, the more it helps."

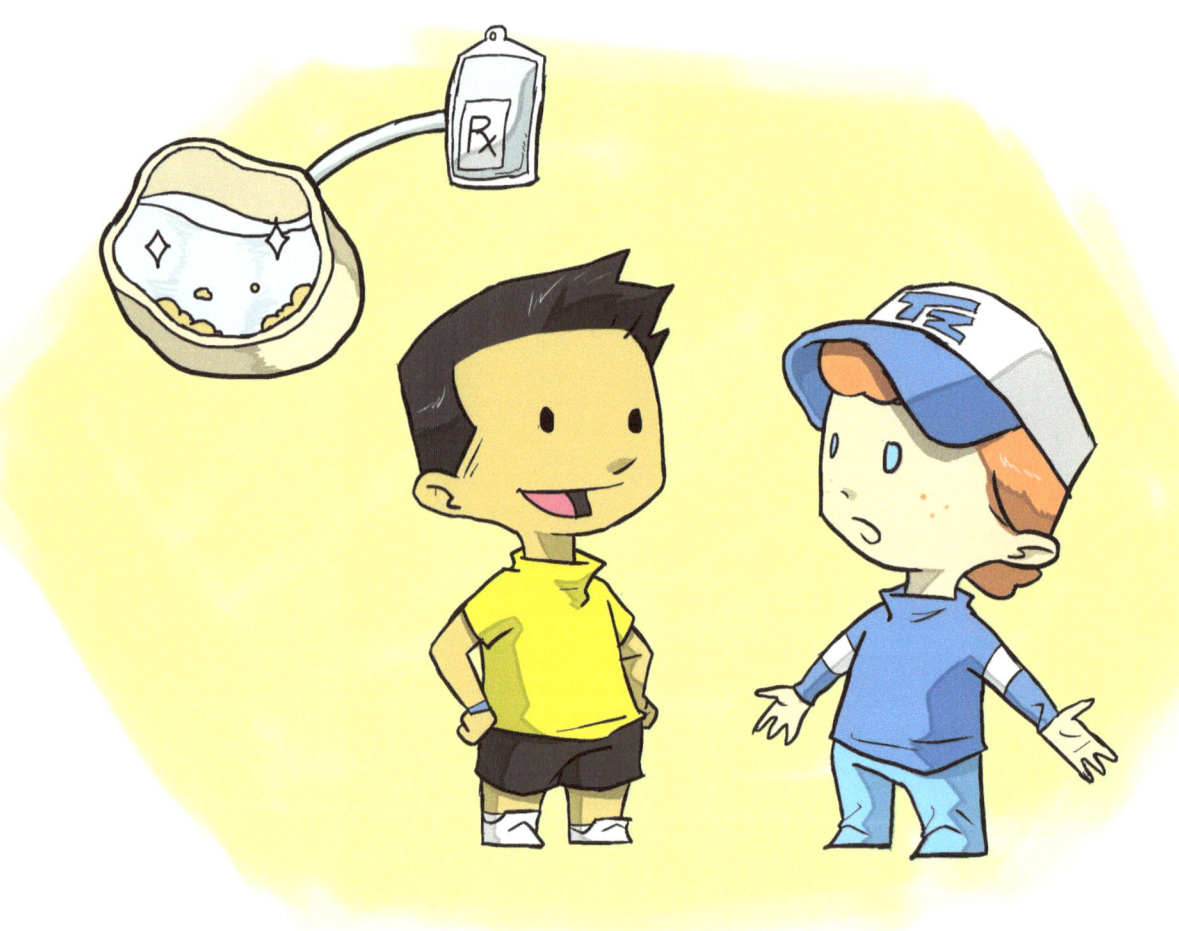

"Hmmmm…" said Robbie, "How often do you get ERT infusions?"

Joe said, "Every other week. It's not a big deal for me. I use a 'no hurt' cream or the cold spray to numb my arm and then they put the medicine in through a tiny needle and 'straw'."

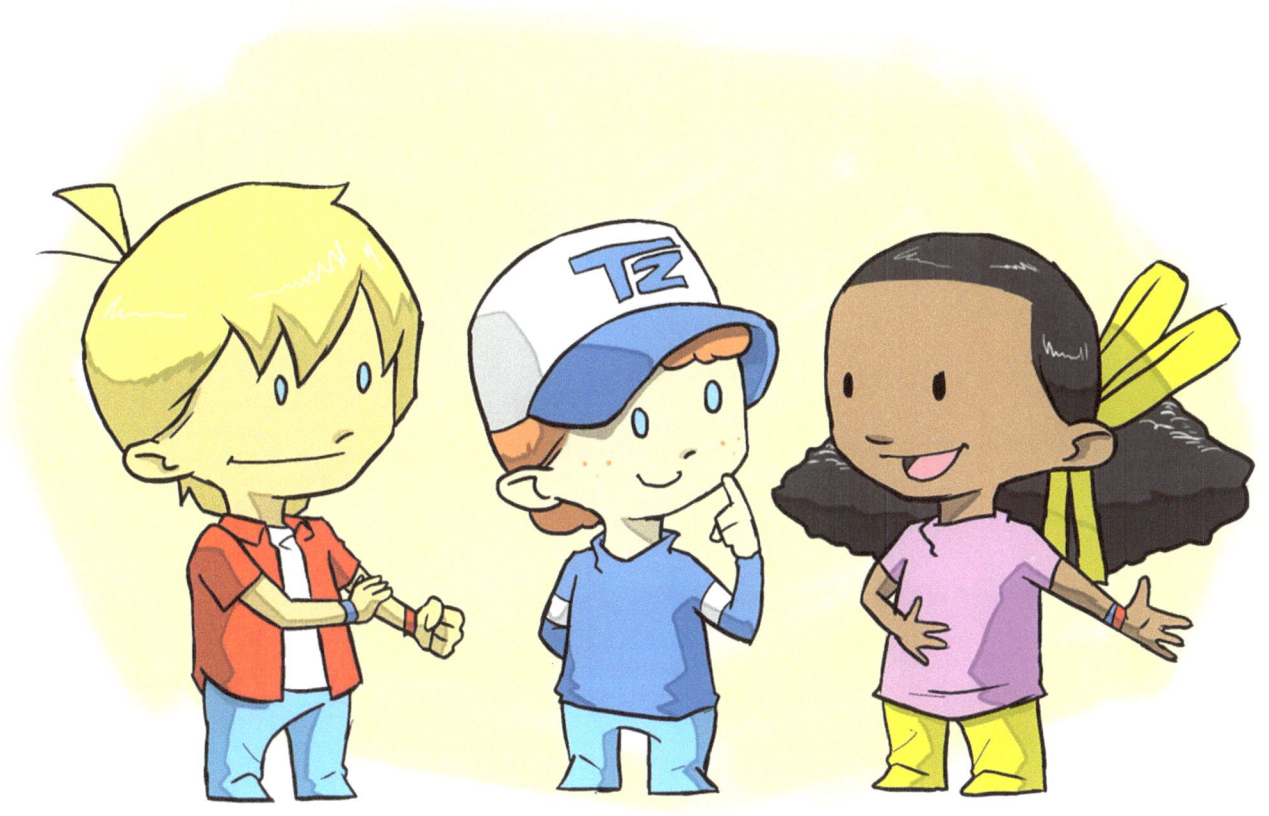

"It was a little scary at first, but the doctor, the nurse, and the genetic counselor explained every step before it happened, so I knew exactly what was coming next. That helped! The other thing that helped was when I got to meet some other kids during my infusions. We talked a lot about infusions in the beginning, but mostly we spent time playing Xbox. Since then some of them have gone to do their infusions at home, but we still email and text."

Dani piped in, "I saw my dad doing infusions before I started. That helped a lot. To me it seems like ERT infusions are a normal thing we do in my family. After I started infusions, it really helped my belly."

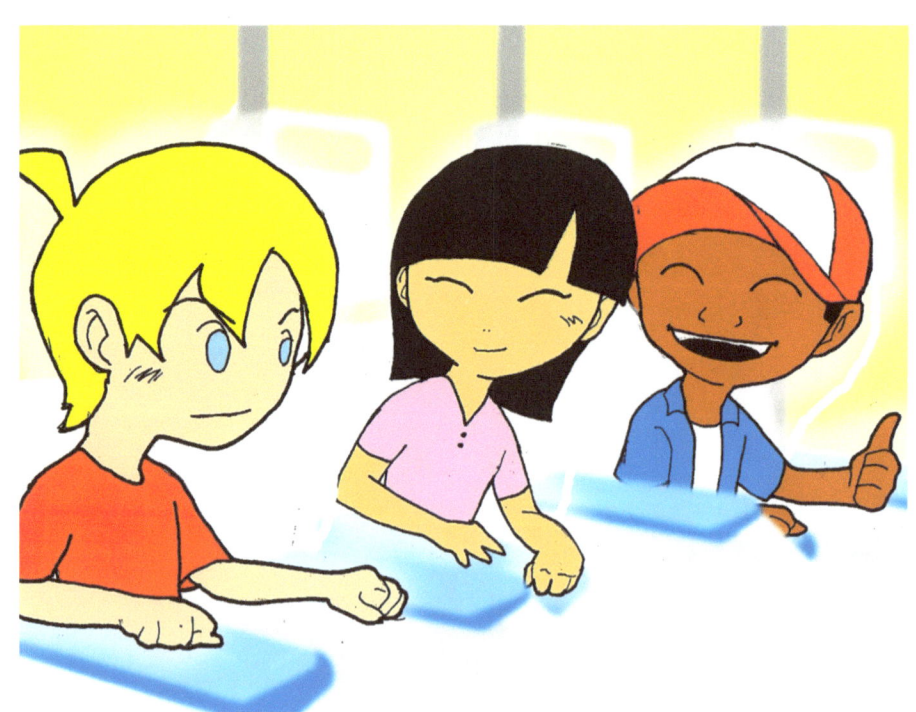

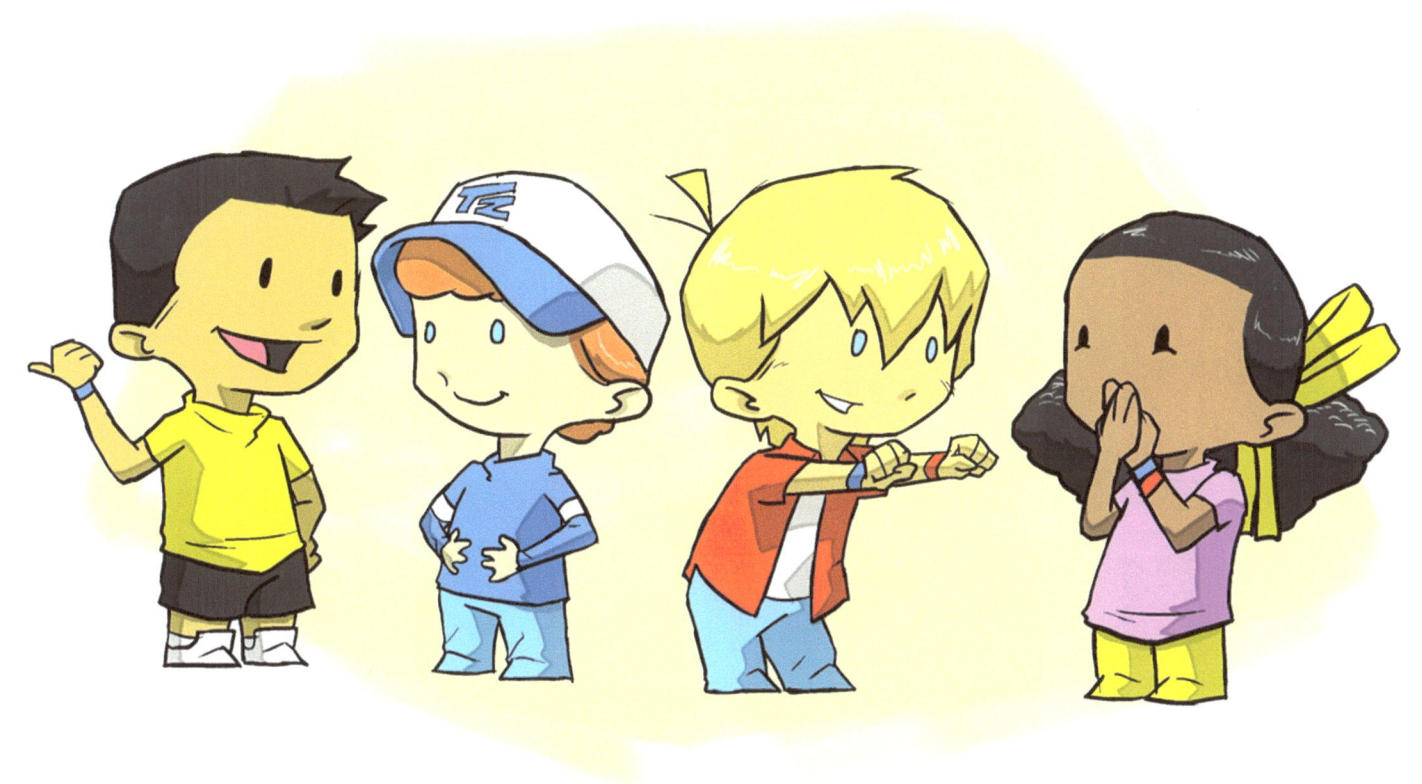

"Speaking of bellies, "said Robbie, "when do we get to eat dinner? I was nervous on the plane so I didn't eat much lunch. I'm starving!"

"Good question," said Joe, "I don't know, should we head back to the cabins and see what the schedule looks like? I know tomorrow night we have Stage Night. Do you guys want to do something together?"

"Sure!" the others agreed.

The four new friends all grinned at each other. They could tell that whatever they did for Stage Night, they would have a great time doing it. This was going to be a great weekend! Even if they never mentioned Fabry disease again, they knew that they could ask each other anything and that'd be ok. They were there to support each other.

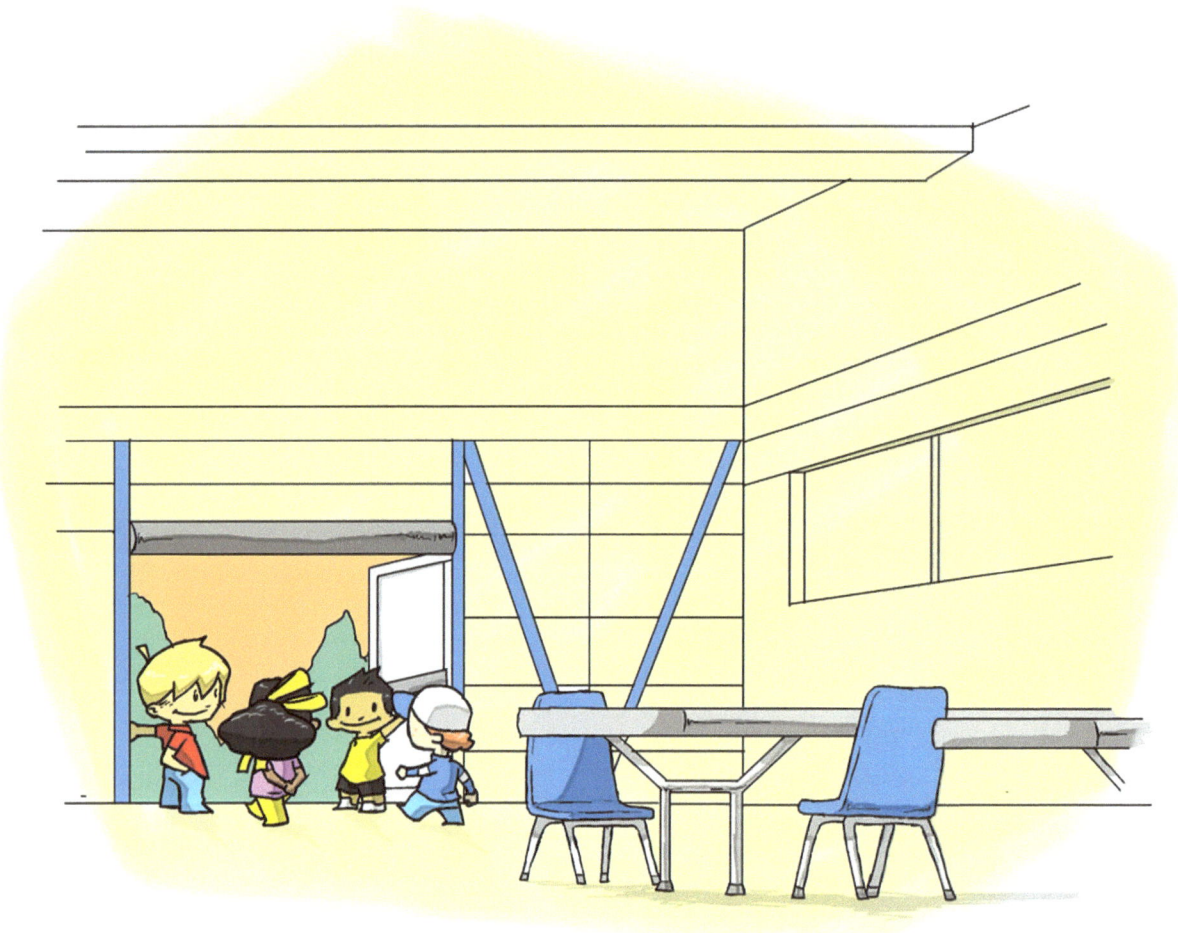

As she returned to her cabin, Dani thought about her bracelets. They made so much sense now: Together they could fight Fabry disease because they were Fabbers helping Fabbers. That's what had just happened here at camp and it was awesome.

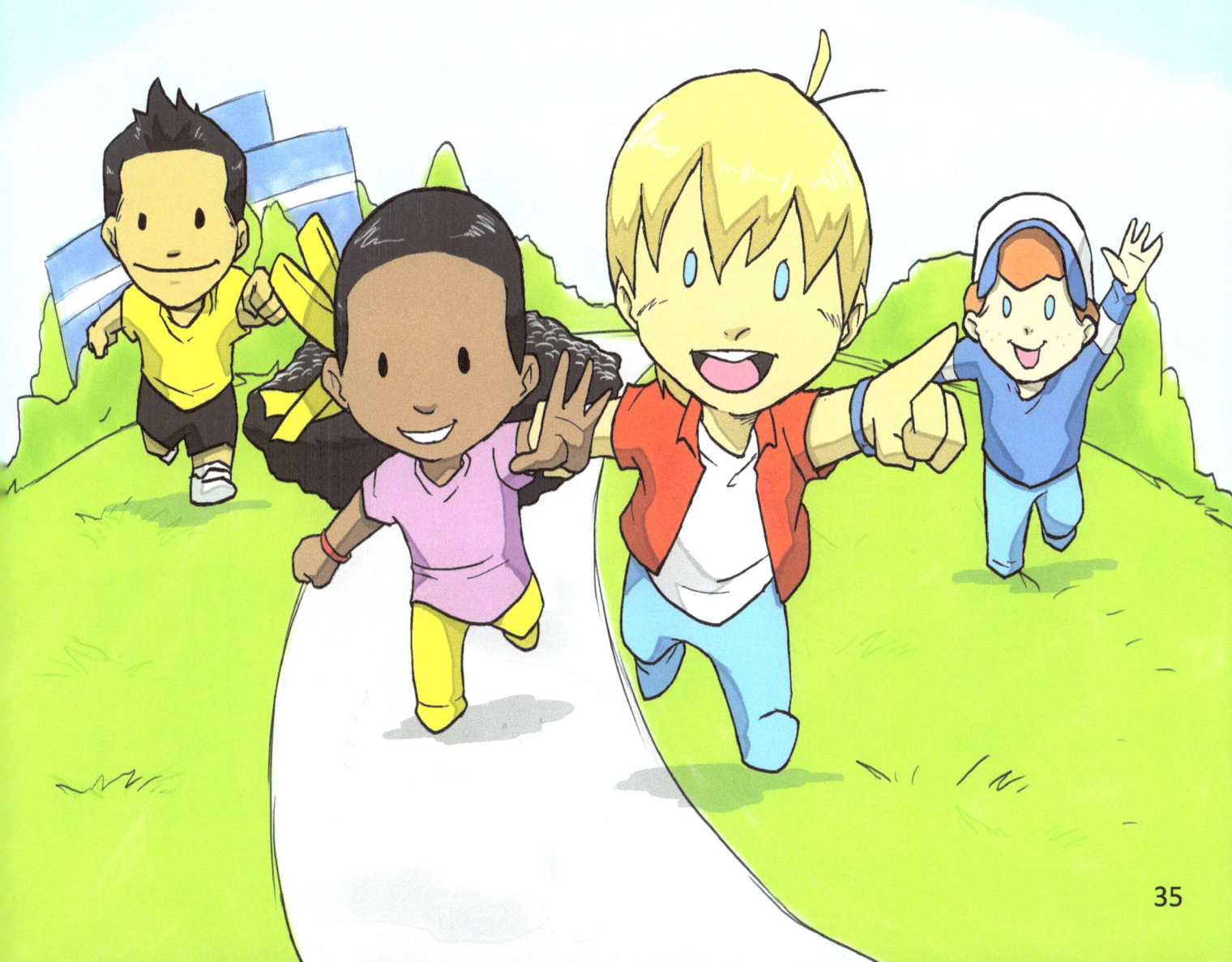

About the Author:

Dawn Laney is an instructor, genetic counselor, and researcher at the Emory Lysosomal Storage Disease Center. She works closely with families affected by Fabry disease and other related conditions. She spends her free time playing with her sons, painting, hiking, reading, and writing children's books.

About the Illustrator:

Michael Johnson is an illustrator and graphic artist living in the Atlanta, Georgia area. His loves are designing video games and staying cool. He knows Dani, Joe, Aaron, and Robbie's pain first hand as he happens to be affected by Fabry disease.

Emory's Lysosomal Storage Disease Center in Atlanta, Georgia provides diagnostic, evaluation, management, and treatment services for patients from all over the United States. The Center is devoted to remaining on the cutting edge of research and treatment providing comprehensive and compassionate care for all of our patients affected by lysosomal storage diseases such as Fabry disease.

To speak with a member of our lysosomal storage disease team, call (404)778-8565 or (800)200-1524 visit our website at http://genetics.emory.edu/LSDC/

Note: This story was developed to help explain Fabry disease and its treatment from the perspective of a preteen or teenager.

Fabry disease is a progressive, inherited metabolic condition caused by a missing or decreased amount of a specific chemical or enzyme known as α-galactosidase A (α-gal A). Typically, α-gal A helps break down a substance called globotriacylceramide, also known as GL-3.

When a person lacks α-galactosidase A, GL-3 builds up in the tissues of the body. The build-up of GL-3 in tissues and blood vessels over time causes problems with the skin, kidneys, stomach, intestines, heart, brain, and nerves. Individuals affected by Fabry disease can have different symptoms than those that described in the book. Common symptoms of Fabry disease in children and teens may include:

- a purplish-pink skin rash (angiokeratoma)
- decreased sweating (Hypohidrosis or anhidrosis)
- gastrointestinal issues including: nausea, vomiting, and alternating diarrhea/constipation
- fatigue
- headaches
- frequent overheating
- sensitivity to extreme temperatures (heat and cold intolerance)
- protein in the urine
- burning or tingling pain in their hands and/or feet (particularly when overheating or sick)

For more information about the symptoms or treatment of Fabry disease, please contact the Emory Lysosomal Storage Disease Center at 800-200-1524 or visit our website at http://genetics.emory.edu/LSDC/ . This book was published with assistance of an educational grant from Genzyme Corporation. Revenue from the sale of this book will be used to support the Emory Lysosomal Storage Disease Center.

www.ingramcontent.com/pod-product-compliance
Lightning Source LLC
Chambersburg PA
CBHW050402180526
45159CB00005B/2119